7 Secrets To Wellness

*Restore your Energy,
Metabolism, and Fatburning
with Doctor-developed
Wellness Secrets*

Dr. Timothy C. Gerhart, D.C., D.A.B.C.I., Dipl. Ac.
**Founder and Director of Renovare Clinic and
Renovare Wellness By Design**

General Notice and Disclaimer

The information and advice given in this book are not intended as substitutes for medical advice or diagnosis. Please consult your health care practitioner if you are experiencing any acute or specific health problems.

While lifestyle, vitamins, minerals, and nutrients do have an important role in preventing and treating sickness and disease, the nutritional supplement products and functional testing described in this book are not intended to diagnose, treat, cure or prevent any disease. The statements in this book have not been evaluated by the Food and Drug Administration.

The patient stories in this book have modified names and details to protect patient privacy. Moreover, each story represents a combination of patient stories to further protect identity.

Copyright 2011 Dr. Timothy C. Gerhart, D.C., D.A.B.C.I., Dipl. Ac.

All rights reserved. This book is protected by the copyright laws of the United States of America and may not be copied or reproduced without the written permission of the author.

ISBN-10: 1466338644

EAN-13: 9781466338647

Table of Contents

INTRODUCTION: VII

SECRET 1:
Fix Your Metabolism So You Lose Weight The Right Way For Good. 1

SECRET 2:
A Balanced, Vibrant Digestive System. 17

SECRET 3:
Secrets to Deep, Restorative Sleep and a Balanced Nervous System. 29

SECRET 4:
Eating Smart. 49

SECRET 5:
Supplementing Smart. 73

SECRET 6:
Exercising Smart. 101

SECRET 7:
Detoxifying Your Body and Emotions. 113

HOW DO I GET STARTED? 127

RESOURCE GUIDE 129

REFERENCES 137

Acknowledgements

This book has been many years in the making. It wasn't until 2 years ago that I started to get serious about writing it. I had been challenged to get it done within a year. It has been said that writing a book is much like having and raising a baby. Lots of work, lots of joy, and a sense of accomplishment are woven with some frustration, weariness, and procrastination – it's taken longer than the year challenge.

This book is really about you. How to help you live with the high level energy, vitality, and Wellness you desire.

It's the stories of my patients from the past 28 years that give me the much needed encouragement and energy to forge ahead. I collect these stories and find much inspiration from the courage and dedication of the remarkable people I have been blessed to work with through the years. It's to you that I dedicate this book of hope and healing.

Many people have been part of making this book happen:

My mother who always believed in my potential and encouraged me until eventually I realized she was right. Her courage to stand against adversity and do what is right has my respect and admiration.

My lovely wife of 28 years, Janet, (where has the time gone?) who is my soul mate, my best friend, confidant and trusted advisor. Without her unwavering support, encouragement, and sacrifice, this book would have never happened and I would not be who I am.

My son, Nate, who has matured into a wonderful, caring, and gifted young man. You have taught me more than you know and I couldn't be prouder of the person you have become.

My dad, Charles, who taught me the value of consistent, determined effort to accomplish what needs to get done. His courage to start businesses and create jobs has been an inspiration.

To Kathy and Marlyn for your support and encouragement on the journey.

To my many mentors and teachers, David McCullum, Will Rodgers, Ron Bettner, Dr. Charles Esch, Dr. Tom Bergmann, Dr. John Allenburg, Dr. Jeffrey Bland, Dr. L. John Faye, Dr. Sandra Spore, Dr. John Amaro, Dr. Micheal Cessna, Dr. Sid Baker, Dr. Brett Saks, Dr. Joseph Mercola, Dr. Perlmutter, Dr. John Duff, Greg Peterson, Gabrielle Loomis, and Debbi Combs.

ACKNOWLEDGEMENTS

My wonderful staff at Renovare who over 28 years of practice have taught me more than a book could hold.

Special thanks to Susan Cali, Jeremy Nye, Richard Taylor and the team at Metagenics for their support, training, resources and kind use of many of the graphics in this book.

Special thanks to Rachelle Tomey, Ryan Frace, and their team for their support, training, and resources.

Special thanks to Christie Howard who has graciously shared her talent and gifting in the cover and graphic design for this book. Much thanks to Chris Mason who shared his gifting in photography for many of the photos in this book.

For Lynn, Bob, Theresa and the others who have graciously helped with proof reading.

And again, my utmost gratitude to the wonderful patients who trust us to be their guide on their journey towards healing and wellness. You provide me with the best training and experience available. As Dr. Brett Saks would say, "Practice certainly graduates the doctor".

Introduction

I am passionate about these 7 Secrets to Wellness – they saved my life.

I lost my health as a young man. I had overworked, overstressed, and overwhelmed my body until something broke deep inside me. I slipped into the depths of terrible, overwhelming fatigue and depression. My motivation, energy, and get-up-and-go got up and went. I ached all over. I suffered with severe gas, bloating, and abdominal cramping. Almost everything I ate made me worse. It got so bad that after 13 hours of sleep, I would wake up exhausted barely able to function. When I walked out of a room, I could not remember who I had just talked to. I kept losing weight. I looked, and felt like I was dying. Without the 7 Secrets to Wellness, I would not be here today.

Now at age 52, after a long journey to regain my health, I am savoring the best health of my adult life. My biologic age is 29 and I look and feel the best in memory. I can work out exercise, travel, work hard, play hard without the limitations of "feeling old or over the hill"

Sadly, I didn't have someone experienced and knowledgeable to guide and help me on my journey back to Wellness. I fought discouragement and despair and understand well those who just give up. I would have given almost anything to have had experienced care, coaching, and encouragement to lighten the load and shorten the journey to Wellness. No one should have to suffer through this alone - without the care, empowerment, and hope that an experienced team of care providers can offer.

My personal struggles and journey have motivated me to pursue continuous and never ending learning to help those struggling to find answers and help. Making the journey back to Wellness as short and easy as possible with lots of caring support is the focus of our team at Renovare and the focus of this book.

Why the name *"Renovare"*?

Renovaré is from Latin "to renew" or "to restore". At Renovare Wellness By Design and Clinic we have made it our passion and purpose to develop the most effective integrated, whole person care to help those suffering with chronic disease so that they can "renew or restore" their health and Wellness.

For the past 28 years, people have been coming to us asking for help with:

- Fatigue, exhaustion, and lack of motivation
- Weight problems and dieting disasters
- Chronic pain problems and migraines
- Chronic anxiety, depression, and mood imbalances
- Hormonal problems
- Sleep problems.
- Cholesterol and triglycerides problems
- Blood sugar problems and insulin resistance
- Diabetes
- Stress management, irritability, and feeling overwhelmed.
- Arthritis, Asthma, Osteoporosis, Colitis, Crohn's, Diverticulitis, GERD
- Alzheimers, Parkinson's, Mysesthenia Gravis, and Brain Fog
- Heart Disease, Chronic Kidney Disease, Thyroid problems
- Scleroderma, Multiple Sclerosis, Lupus, Sjogren's, Rheumatoid Arthritis, and many of the other 180+ autoimmune diseases
- Returning to an active lifestyle
- Optimizing their health and staying well throughout their lifespan

Mary's Story

Mary came to our clinic recently and shared her story. She had developed sores on her inner ankle that progressed to an open wound. Since she didn't have insurance, she tried home treatments – no luck.

Next, she went to a medical physician (trained in acute disease care). He ran tests and tried antibiotics – no improvement. The wound progressed to a deep pocket – you could insert 3 fingers into it! Her MD referred her to a specialist and again more (acute care) tests – could not figure it out. Guessed at a diagnosis and sent her to yet another specialist. More (acute care) tests and not sure what it is.

Mary had now burned through over $10,000.00 of her precious savings with no answers and little help! She is faced with losing her home and declaring bankruptcy with her medical bills overwhelming her limited savings.

Sadly, I hear this type of story time after time.

What Went Wrong with our Medical Disease Care System for Mary?

Almost 80% or our health care problems in America are now <u>CHRONIC disease care problems. Guess what kind of training our medical physicians in America receive? That's right, virtually no training for CHRONIC disease. Chronic diseases are those that last over 90 days.</u>

Doctors are trained in medical schools in America to treat acute diseases (last less than 90 days) like:

- Severe infections
- Broken bones
- Heart Attacks,
- Severe blood loss
- Strokes
- Trauma, wounds, and life-threatening crises

TV shows like E.R. portray the heroic efforts of our medical professionals saving lives with amazing trauma care surgery and miraculous medications.

Guess what kind of condition Mary had? She was suffering with a chronic autoimmune disease for which her doctors had little training or even the tools to help her.

Repeat this for almost 80% of our health problems - chronic disease - and we have an expensive mess!

This helps to explain how we spend more money per person (by far) on health care than any country on the planet and have a dismal, terrible, embarrassing Health System Ranking of 37th by the World Health Organization. We are doing so poorly that even countries like Columbia and Costa Rica beat us in the ranking.[1]

So What Is Wrong With Our Medical Training?

Halstead Holman, MD. Dean Emeritus of Stanford School of Medicine has written and published articles in medical journals such as the one below published in the *Journal of the American Medical Association*. (2)

Chronic Disease—The Need for a New Clinical Education

"It is axiomatic that medical education should prepare students well for the clinical problems they will face in their future practice. However, that is not happening for the most prevalent problem in health care today: chronic disease."

---

1 A full listing of references is available in reference section at end of this book.

"The inadequacy of clinical education is a consequence of the failure of health care and medical education to adapt to 2 related transformations in the past 50 years that are central to good health care today. In the first, chronic disease replaced acute disease as the dominant health problem. Chronic disease is now the principal cause of disability and use of health services and consumes 78% of health expenditures. In the second, chronic disease dramatically transformed the role of the patient."

"The differences between acute and chronic disease are substantial. Acute disease is episodic. The patient is usually inexperienced and passive while the physician administers treatment." see the full text of the article at reference [2]

Dr. Halstead writes that we need a new medical training approach for physicians to help those with chronic (long-standing) health problems. The acute care (emergency-room) model of health care in ineffective and far too costly for most of our chronic disease problems.

In the book, "Living a Healthy Life With Chronic Conditions", co-written by Dr. Halstead, the approach is to teach people to manage their chronic disease – whether it be heart disease, diabetes, arthritis, or asthma.

The book includes a nice chart contrasting the different care approaches. I modified and expanded the chart to create the chart below:

Medical Care Approaches

	ACUTE DISEASE:	CHRONIC DISEASE:
Beginning	• Rapid	• Gradual
Cause	• Often just one	• Many roots
Duration	• Short	• Long-term
Diagnosis	• Usually accurate	• Often uncertain
Testing (Medical)	• Often decisive	• Often limited value
Testing (LifeStyle)	• Not applicable	• Whole person
Medical Treatment	• Cure common	• Cure rare (drug reactions)
Lifestyle Treatment	• Not applicable	• Often helpful/treat roots
Doctor/Team	• Give treatment	• Listen, empower, coach
Patient Role	• Follow orders	• Responsible for Life change
Care Process	• Brief - prescribe	• Extended relationship-based
	• Treat disease	• Treat whole person

---

2 JAMA 2004;292(9):1057-1059 Halsted Holman, MD Author Affiliation: Stanford University, School of Medicine, Palo Alto, Calif.

Since our medical providers are trained in only the acute care approach, they tend to view each patient through the lens of the acute care model. This is great for acute care problems, but what about chronic disease?

If the only tool you have is a hammer (acute care) you tend to see every problem as a nail. Far too often, the "hammer" of acute care treatment with powerful drugs and surgeries is used for chronic disease. This is like using a hammer to loosen a delicate Phillips-head screw - not effective and likely to cause more harm than good.

Our body is an amazingly complex, delicate biologic system. With chronic disease, we need sensitive treatment approaches to help shift this delicate system towards balance and Wellness. Using powerful drugs is like trying to use a hammer to kill a fly on a window. The heavy hammer is awkward and likely to miss – and the window pane is likely to suffer more harm than help.

Acute care "hammers" are simply the wrong tool for the job.

Another Problem is That We Expect our Medical Doctors to be Experts in Everything

Dr. Alex Vasquez, a brilliant lecturer, author, and "triple Doc" - Chiropractic physician degree, Naturopathic Medical degree, and now a Osteopathic Medical degree - was describing his recent experience at a highly rated medical school as a 4th year medical student. His medical school professor came into the class and stated that, "Diet, nutrition, and lifestyle are profoundly important in health and disease".

Then silence.

His professor then moved on to the next subject regarding pharmacology (study of drugs). That was the extent of his training regarding diet, lifestyle and nutrition in Medical School.

With few exceptions, my medical physician colleagues tell me they got "zippo, nada, nothing" regarding effective training in diet, nutrition, vitamins, or lifestyle. Expecting our medical physicians to be experts in these areas is unrealistic – they are experts in pharmacology - as we need them to be.

My MD colleagues and friends tell me that they often feel frustrated and ill-equipped for the chronic disease patients they see – they dread it, but are expected by their employers and insurance contracts to write a prescription and move on.

This helps to explain why medical providers sometimes do things that don't make sense (and harm more than help) for those who struggle with a list of chronic diseases.

With few exceptions, my medical colleagues are highly trained, dedicated, caring professionals who provide the essential acute care when we need it. Asking these medical professionals to treat chronic disease without the needed training or tools isn't fair to them or to their patients. Would you expect your dentist to do your dental care with gardening tools?

The far too few MD's who do have training and experience in treating chronic disease have pursued this training on their own – often at great expense and risk of criticism from their peers. I applaud these courageous pioneers who are way ahead of the curve. Another way to look at it is:

Acute Care Approach

- One problem
- One cause
- One treatment

This is called linear thinking. This approach should be limited to acute care problems. The diagram below shows why this works so poorly for chronic care problems:

Non-Functional Care Model:

Symptom ➡ Treatment

In contrast, a Functional Care model that works really well for most chronic care problems looks like:

Functional Care Model:

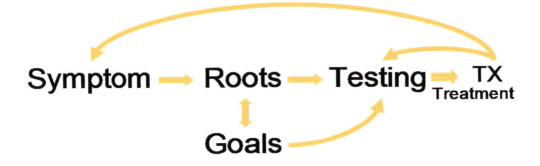

The Functional Care Model diagram shows the Renovare approach we have found effective for treating patients suffering with chronic disease.

At Renovare, we don't seek to treat or cure chronic disease. For someone with Asthma, Arthritis, or Parkinson's Disease, we are more interested in the person with the disease than the name of the disease.

For Parkinson's, as with most chronic diseases, if you have one hundred people diagnosed with Parkinson's, you have 100 different diseases. Everyone is different with unique genetics, a unique environment and LifeStyle, and a unique manifestation of their body imbalance or disease.

We work to support our Natural healing process so we move "up the curve" toward Wellness as the graphic below shows:

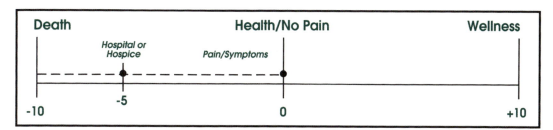

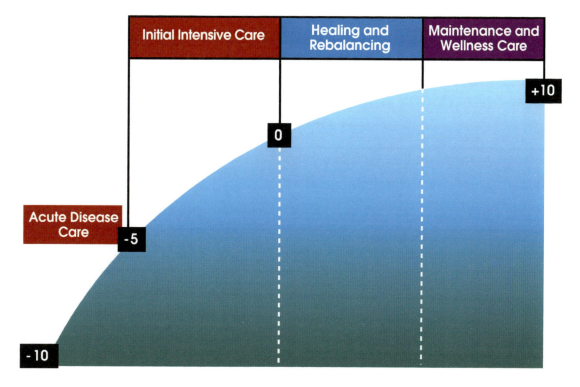

Many think that the absence of pain equals being well — not true. Being pain-free is just level 0. Imagine if you only decided to brush your teeth or visit your dentist when your teeth hurt — that would be neglect. Moving to high level Wellness – well above level 0 - is our best insurance against disease and sickness.

In our care approach at Renovare, we move beyond the label or diagnosis and start asking questions like:
- How did your chronic degenerative disease start and progress over the years?
- What kind of LifeStyle imbalances, toxic exposure, excessive toxic stress contributed to your downward slide?
- What are the likely roots (plural) behind the development of your diseases?
- What have you been missing to support your Natural Healing Response?

In short, "Dis-ease" is really a body out of balance and a LifeStyle that does not fit our genetic needs.

I remember Dr. Sidney Baker M.D. saying, "To get well, get rid of the bad stuff and add the good stuff".

So Why Read This Book?

Here are some reasons:
- I am sick and tired of being sick and tired.
- I have suffered far too long with:
    - Fatigue – my energy and stamina are plunging and getting worse.
    - Gaining fat and nothing works anymore to lose it and keep it off.
    - Pain! I hurt too much and suffer with chronic inflammation that bounces from one body part to another.
    - Sleep problems – it's terrible and I dread getting up in the morning.
    - Digestive problems – my bowels move too often or not enough. I suffer gas, bloating, and food reactions. I can't enjoy eating anymore.
    - Brain Fog! I can't remember, focus, concentrate like I used to.
    - Emotional Roller coaster – up, down, just can't find a peaceful balance.
    - Hormones – always been off or went through a stressful time and just not re-balancing again.
    - STRESS! I can't handle it anymore and struggle with anxiety and worry I can't seem to control.
    - I look and feel old – I think young, just my body is not cooperating.
    - I feel like I turned 30, or 40, or 50 and started to fall apart. I am sliding and dread what I will be like in 10 years if I don't get help – and soon!

- I have been unwell too long and feel ready to give up. I despair of ever finding help.
- I am sick of just taking pills to cover up my symptoms. I want answers to what is the root of my problems and how to get well.

My primary care provider or MD hasn't told me about this, why should I believe it?

Therapeutic LifeStyle Change(TLC) is now the recognized standard of care for chronic disease.

In 2004, in the highly respected medical journal Circulation (3), the American Heart Association, American Diabetes Association, and the American Cancer Society jointly published a landmark article in which they state that Therapeutic Lifestyle Change is the "first line of therapy" for most chronic disease.

Therapeutic Lifestyle Change (TLC)

RECOMMENDED BY:
- National Institutes of Health
- American Heart Association
- American Cancer Society
- American Diabetes Association
- Arthritis Foundation
- North American Menopause Society

...and many others as a "first line" treatment for conditions most doctors see every day.

CONDITIONS:
- High Cholesterol
- High Blood Pressure
- High Blood Sugar and/or Diabetes
- Heart Disease
- Osteoporosis
- Metabolic Syndrome
- Menopausal Symptoms
- Many Others

In other words, for most chronic disease, the place to start is LifeStyle change, not just popping a pill.

When I graduated from Northwestern College of Chiropractic in 1983, I had a great foundation in natural healing, clinical nutrition, healthy lifestyle and more. I also realized that in many ways I knew just enough to get started - or just enough to be dangerous. My youth and inexperience were an interesting combination.

Over the past 28 years I have been blessed to receive extensive advanced training from Dr. Jeffrey Bland, PhD, the Father of Functional Medicine, and many others. Traveling the country attending seminars from many of the top experts in the field became an addiction for me. I invested in the extensive, multi-year post-graduate training to become a board-certified Chiropractic Internist. This was followed by training to become a Diplomate of the International Academy of Medical Acupuncture.

My ongoing educational process and clinical experience have taught me a humbling sense of how much I don't know. Each person is genetically unique with a unique life experience and LifeStyle choices. The statistical average human doesn't exist – at least I haven't met one in the past 28 years. Research and probabilities only go so far – they are of very limited value as I listen to the person sitting beside me in our clinic with their unique history, genetics, personality, and desires. I have come to understand there is much more I don't know than what I do know regarding the person coming to me for help.

Because of this realization, I have learned to profoundly value listening to the person who has been living in their own body. The most powerful step to helping someone is to really, really, really listen to their story of how they got to where they are, ask guiding questions to learn clues as to why they have their problems, and seek to understand the picture their symptoms create. Then, most importantly, unravel the likely roots or causes of their problems.

Integrating, or putting together all of the pieces of the puzzle of how someone became sick and unwell is the first step.

The next, even more challenging step, is delivering the integrated or unified care process to effectively deal with each "root" or cause of the long list of health problems. One doctor told me the reason he got into *wholistic* medicine is that his patients kept coming to him with a *whole* long list of health problems.

This means providing care and providing the teaching and empowering each person needs to progress on their healing journey and create a LifeStyle that fits their unique needs and desires. For most this includes the 7 Secrets to Wellness to follow through this book.

The last step, is building a team of passionate, committed professionals who put patient care first and live out "relationship is everything". I am grateful and blessed to work with such a team.

Who is Dr. Gerhart?

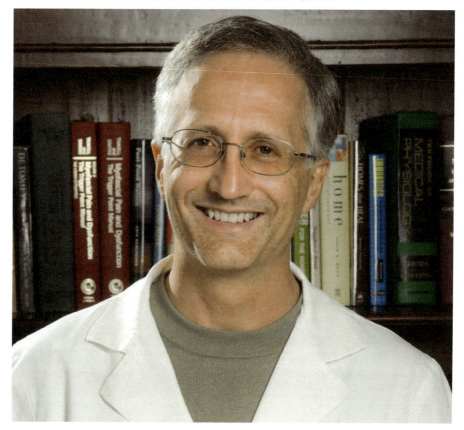

Hello I am Dr. Timothy C. Gerhart, D.C., D.A.B.C.I., Dipl. Ac.

I am a Board-certified Chiropractic Internist and Chiropractic Physician utilizing a natural LifeStyle-based approach that works to help each patient reach their individual goals. I have advanced training and extensive experience in helping patients as well as teaching other physicians in:

- Blood Laboratory Testing
- Acupuncture and energy therapies
- Nutritional supplements, herbs, homeopathic remedies
- Gentle adjustments of spine, foot, ankle, knee, wrist, elbow, shoulder and jaw joints
- Frequency Specific Microcurrent (FSM) and low-level laser for healing, inflammation, and pain relief
- Hormone, Vitamin, and Mineral testing
- Lab evaluation of cellular energetics underlying fatigue and chronic illness
- Answering some of the "Why" questions behind pain, illness and un-wellness

- Adhesion/scar tissue release techniques.
- Working with Dental, Medical, and other care providers

My background:

- A National Merit Scholar at the University of North Dakota and graduated at the top of my class from Northwestern College of Chiropractic (now Northwestern University of Health Sciences) in 1983.
- A registered acupuncturist with extensive training and experience in bioelectric testing and treatment.
- Diplomate status (highest level of training) with the International Academy of Medical Acupuncture.
- Wrote and taught the post-graduate course in Laboratory Diagnostics for the American Board of Chiropractic Internists through National College of Chiropractic (now National University of Health Sciences).
- Laboratory test interpretation computer software designer and developer
- Diplomate of the American Board of Chiropractic Internists
- Past president of the Midwest Chiropractic Internists Association
- Member of the American Chiropractic Association Council on Diagnosis and Internal Disorders.
- Member of the Arizona Chiropractic Association
- Past member and presenter for the Institute of Functional Medicine
- 2000 recipient of the Dr. Bill Nelson Award for Advancing Excellence in Patient Care and Physician Education by the American Chiropractic Association Council on Family Practice
- Founder of Renovare Institute which trains Chiropractic, Medical, Naturopathic, and Osteopathic physicians, and LifeStyle Coaches in LifeStyle Healing
- Certified in Therapeutic Lifestyle Change and a Center of Clinical Excellence for First Line Therapy

My staff and I have been helping patients since 1983 – 21 years in Minnesota and the past 9 years in Arizona.

We especially delight in helping those who have fallen through the cracks of our disease care system by restoring hope for healing – naturally!

Now, almost 28 years later, my many patients, mentors, teachers, and staff have taught me:

- Our health is mostly the result of our choices. We are responsible for our current level of health.
- Our LifeStyle mostly and our genetics to a lesser degree determine our level of Wellness.
- We have a fantastic (almost unbelievable) self-healing ability – it's almost never too late.
- Getting well involves getting rid of enough of the "bad stuff", and adding in enough of the needed "good stuff".
- Asking "Why" and persistently pursuing answers is key to getting to the "roots" of our health problems.
- Putting together (Integrating) the pieces of our puzzle so we can start healing is far more important than just labeling our condition and using the "pill for each ill" approach.
- **Healing is all about relationships** – relationship with ourselves, family, friends, and get this – health care providers/trusted resources/coaches/mentors.
- A few basic changes go a long way – *it is about progress, not perfection*.
- Everyone is unique – one size does NOT fit all.
- Most of us need someone with experience and training to guide, encourage, and measure our progress. Change takes time and without help, it's too easy to get sidetracked or discouraged and give up.
- We are responsible for our own journey towards Wellness – our team of care providers serve as our guides, coaches, and support.
- Expecting a doctor or care provider to be responsible for your long-term health is dysfunctional – you are responsible for your own health journey.

My staff and I have had the immense satisfaction and fulfillment of sharing in the journeys of many in which almost everyone experiences improvement – most substantial – as long as they cooperate and continue their needed LifeStyle changes.

Join us as we share our stories and insights through the 7 Secrets to Wellness. We wish you only the very best on your journey toward the high level energy, vitality, and Wellness you desire.

Secret 1

FIX YOUR METABOLISM SO YOU LOSE WEIGHT THE RIGHT WAY FOR GOOD

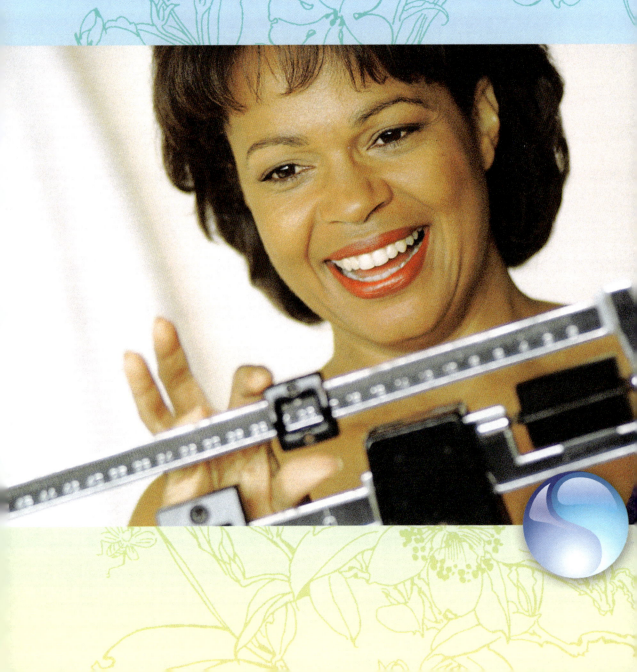

Chapter 1 Snapshot

- Have you suffered through diet after diet with repeated failures?
- Have you gained and lost the same 30 pounds too many times to remember?
- Are you ready to do it right so that you NEVER need to DIET again?

Here is what you need to know:

- The problem isn't you
- Diets don't work – they lead to muscle loss and damaged metabolism
- Repairing your metabolism and creating a LifeStyle that fits your unique genetic needs is the only way to long-term success
- Gaining muscle and metabolic tissue leads to easy fat loss
- Instead of dieting, it is essential to "feed" your metabolism so that you gain muscle and boost your metabolism
- We need all of the Secrets to Wellness working for our metabolism to work well
  - Our **Digestive** system must be balanced and healthy
  - Our **Nervous** system must be balanced and peaceful. We must **Sleep** well.
  - We must be **Eating Smart** to fit our metabolism
  - We must be **Supplementing Smart** to fit our unique genetic and LifeStyle needs
  - We must be **Exercising Smart** to fit our needs – and building muscle and body cell mass
  - We must be **Detoxifying** our emotions and our body for our metabolism to work well

Emma's Story

Emma came to us after years of failing at diet after diet. She was frustrated and ready to give up. She was 5'6" tall, age 32, and weighed 219 lbs. She hated the way she looked and felt.

We started our first consult with the magic question, "In a perfect world in which you could have ANYTHING you wanted regarding your health – no limitations – what would be at the top of your list?" Predictably, she said "Weight Loss".

I asked Emma, "Do you really want to lose <u>weight?</u>"

I then showed her this diagram:

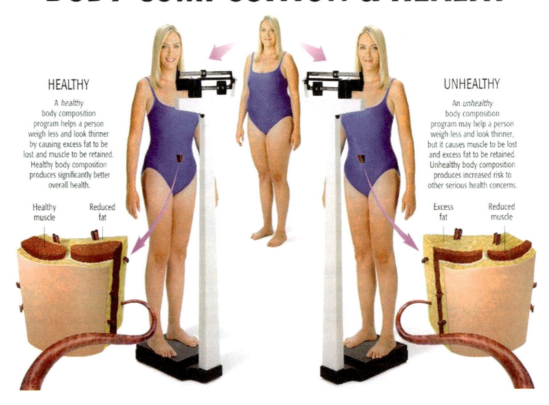

Graphic kindly provided by Metagenics

The woman on the left lost only the "yellow stuff"- fat- and kept her precious muscle vital to her metabolism.

The woman on the right lost only the "red stuff" – muscle – and damaged her metabolism in the process.

What's the Result?

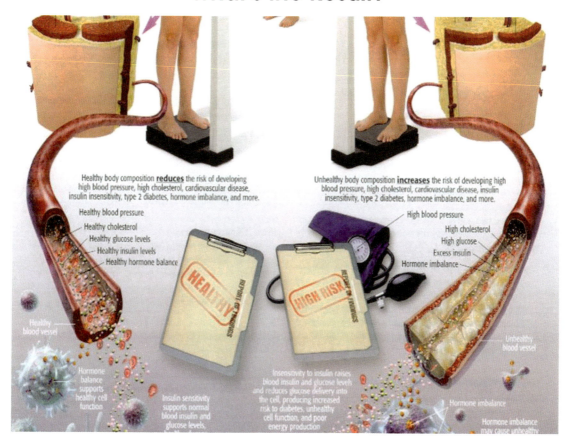

Graphic kindly provided by Metagenics

The woman on the right lost muscle, damaged her metabolism, increased inflammation, and messed up her blood sugar, insulin, and hormone balance. When she went off this disastrous, deprivation diet, she gained back all the weight plus some. Next time she tries to "diet" it will be even harder until eventually, dieting and exercise won't work.

When we tested Emma, we found a body fat of 54% and body cell mass (muscle and organ tissue that burn calories and make up our metabolic tissue) of just 19.8%. She had severely damaged her metabolism with her repeated dieting and damaging lifestyle.

I told Emma, "You are not so much overweight as you are *underlean*. You don't have one ounce of weight (as muscle) you can afford to lose! The thinking that got you into your current mess is not the thinking that can solve it."

Do you want to be successful? You must change your focus. How about a goal of: **Become lean and fit through repairing my metabolism so that I gain muscle and lose fat easily so that I look and feel good about myself.**

"Can my metabolism be repaired after all the damage I have caused?" asked Emma.

With few exceptions, the answer is yes. If the winner of our recent "Greatest Loser" contest, Jubie Hughes, could turn around her damaged metabolism at age 82 and win the contest over contestants less than half her age, almost anybody can do it. Here is what you need to know:

Repairing Your Metabolism

Overview:

1. Healthy, balanced metabolism results in lots of energy, vibrant youthfulness even as we age, and staying lean and trim easily.

2. Damaged metabolism results in lower energy and gaining weight more and more easily in spite of diets, exercise, and LOTS of effort to lose weight.

3. Diets may help lose weight – esp. when younger – but often result in losing muscle, gaining fat, and damaging your metabolism.

4. Your metabolism – for the most part – equals your muscle. Losing muscle = damaging your metabolism.

5. Weight loss can be damaging and destructive to your metabolism and health unless you are carefully *measuring* your muscle gain and fat loss.

6. Diets typically fail, instead a LifeStyle that supports metabolism repair, muscle gain and fat loss is vitally important for success that lasts.

7. The best tool, in my 28 years of experience, to assess your metabolism, toxicity, muscle mass, and fat mass is whole body bioimpedance. At Renovare, we refer to this as our Body Composition and Metabolism Assessment.

8. Standing on a bioimpedance scale at a gym only measures your legs and pelvic area. Holding onto a bioimpedance device with your hands only measures your arm and chest area.

9. To be effective with bioimpedance, we need to measure from your wrist/hand area to your foot/ankle area with ECG electrodes so we measure *your whole body* composition. Combining this with sophisticated, research-supported software and the clinical experience to interpret your results is what it takes to do it right.

Why is Your Metabolism Such a Big Deal?

When your metabolism is "supercharged" you can eat and eat (the right food to fuel your needs of course) and stay lean, fit, and full of energy! You never need to diet. Instead you eat 5 times or more per day to build muscle and fuel your metabolism. You look and feel great – even as you get older – this is successful aging!

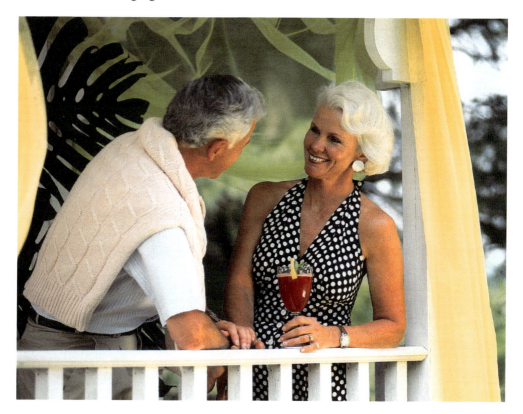

What is Metabolism?

It is converting food (and oxygen) to energy (as ATP and heat). This process is also called respiration as in diagram below:

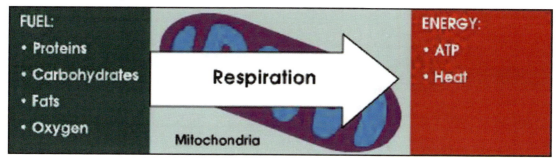

Where Does Metabolism Happen?

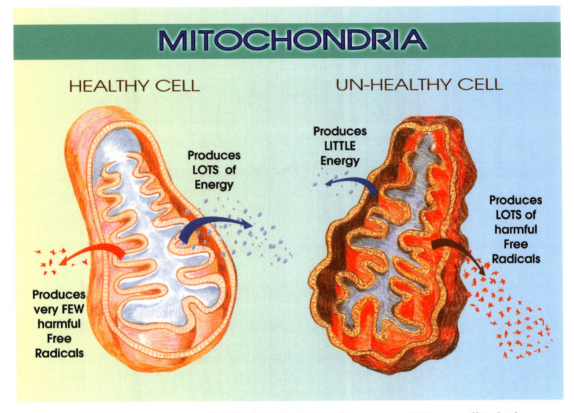

These energy "factories" are in each cell of our body. We have up to 2000 per cell in high energy cells like heart muscle cells and neurons in our brain. They are the engines where the vast majority of our metabolism or energy production occurs. When healthy, 10% of our body weight is our mitochondria and they generate our body weight daily in ATP – the fuel that powers us. The ATP molecule recycles 1000 -1500X per day to accomplish this.

Think of the "3M's":

1. Metabolism
2. Mitochondria
3. Muscle

They are all linked. If you want better metabolism, build muscle and mitochondria.

What Does Our Metabolism Look Like?

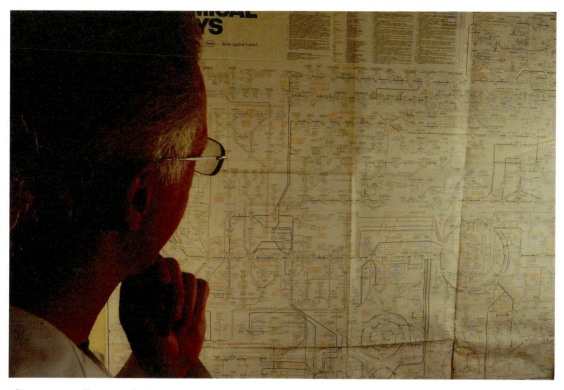

This is a small part of the complex biochemistry of cellular metabolism. With our metabolic "machinery" so intricate and complicated, do we really want to fuel it with junk food or damage it with silly LifeStyle choices?

So What Damages Our Metabolism?

Dieting! We have an irrational obsession with "losing weight" and dieting! We lose and then gain back even more. We endure failure after failure and begin to lose hope. Sometimes we even blame ourselves, "I have no self control and I AM A FAILURE".

**Good news is that the problem isn't you!
Dieting just doesn't work.**

Why?

Diets Don't Work

1. Regular dieting shown to predict <u>**weight gain** and increased risk of chronic disease.</u> [1]
2. "Yo-Yo" dieting linked to increased risk of cardiovascular disease, stroke, diabetes, and immune dysfunction.[2]

The real problem with deprivation dieting is that it damages our metabolism!

How Do I Know If My Metabolism Is Damaged?

1. Low energy, low stamina
2. Hormonal imbalances – esp. if increased belly fat
3. Accelerated aging
4. Lab test findings like elevated cholesterol, triglycerides, or blood glucose
5. Body Composition and Metabolism (BCM) assessment
6. Failure to respond to exercise and eating smart

---

[1] *AM Psycol, 2007 April 62(3); 220-33*
[2] *www.physorg.com/news94906931.html*

So How Do We Measure Our Metabolism?

The Body **Composition and Metabolism Assessment (BCM)** is one of my favorite tools to assess your metabolism, muscle mass, and fat mass. It is safe, painless, accurate, and ultra budget-friendly. The assessment utilizes whole body bioimpedence with ECG electrodes on your wrist, hand, foot and ankle to get your results. A test sample looks like:

Name :	Emma Damaged Metabolism	ID # :	
Gender :	Female	Height :	56 in
Age :	32	Current Weight :	219 lb

Study date :	08/22/2011 4:10:58 PM	Report date 08/22/2011	4:11:06 PM
Current weight :	219 lb	BMI :	49.10
Measured Resistance :	330 ohms	Measured Reactance :	34 ohms
Calculated Impedance :	331.7 ohms	Phase Angle :	5.9 degrees
Parallel Resistance :	333.5 ohms	Parallel Capacitance :	983 pf
Impedance Index :	1176.2	Ideal weight :	80.0 lb
Equation Set :	Cyprus/FNA		
Test Comments :			

Predicted results based on bioelectrical impedance analysis

FLUID ASSESSMENT	Results	Target range	Percent of actual	Comment
Total Body Water	38.7 L	15.0 - 19.4 Liters	38.9 % (WT)	*
Intracellular Water	18.0 L	9.0 - 11.2 Liters	46.4 % (TBW)	*
Extracellular Water	20.7 L	6.0 - 8.2 Liters	53.6 % (TBW)	*
NUTRITION ASSESSMENT				
Basal Metabolism	1370 Kcals			
Body Cell Mass	43.4 lb	20.5 - 28.5 lb	19.8 % (WT)	*
Extracellular Mass	56.7 lb	34.2 - 42.2 lb	25.9 % (WT)	*
Fat Free Mass (FFM)	100.1 lb	60.7 - 64.7 lb	45.7 % (WT)	*
Fat Mass	118.9 lb	15.3 - 19.3 lb	54.3 % (WT)	*

This Is What the Results Mean

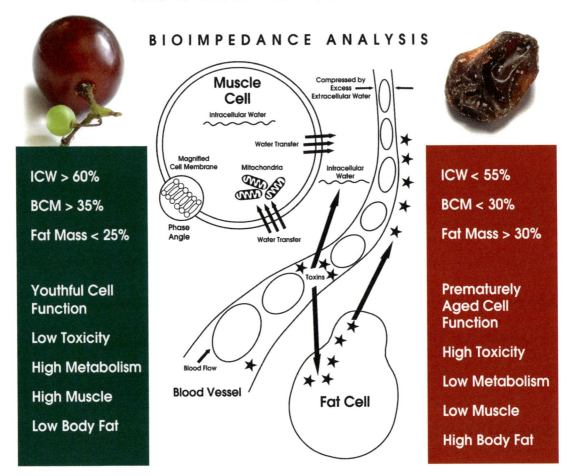

The three most important numbers on your test results are:

1. **ICW = Intracellular water.** This reflects your metabolism and how well your mitochondria (cell energy factories) generate ATP (cell energy) to power the pumps that move nutrients and water into your cells and power the detoxification pathways (Chapter 7) to process and move toxins out of your cells. When this works well, your cells are plump, happy, and youthful – and you are thin, fit, and energetic. When this works poorly, your cells are shriveled (raisin-like), sickly, and toxic – and you are fat, bloated, and toxic.

2. **BCM = Body Cell Mass** (Muscle and Organ tissue rich in mitochondria that power your metabolism). When you are repairing your metabolism, this goes up. This is the best measurement of healthy aging. When you lose weight, you must guard against losing this!

3. **Fat Mass = stored energy** at 3500 calories per pound of stored fat. Fat is not bad, it is stored energy. Rather than get upset with our fat, let's ask why we aren't

burning it. If you have excessive body fat, it is a metabolism problem, not a fat problem. When you are successfully repairing your metabolism, you lose only fat and maintain your precious muscle, mitochondria and metabolic tissue.

By doing follow-up Body Composition and Metabolism Assessments at intervals of 2-4 weeks during a Metabolism Repair program, we can assess your progress, what you are losing, and if you are becoming toxic because of fat loss.

Another tool is the "LifeStyle Score" which you can take to both assess your current LifeStyle Score and improvement at 2 or 4 week intervals. Improvements in your energy level and your waist to hip ratio are especially important signs of improving metabolism. The LifeStyle score is in the Reference Guide at the end of this book.

Why Would Fat Loss Create Problems?

What is stored in our body fat? How about some of the most toxic, nasty chemicals on the planet! (3)

The charts below document some of the toxins found on extensive testing of 9 diverse participants (including PBS journalist Bill Moyers) by Mount Sinai School of Medicine.(4)

167 Compounds from seven chemical groups were found in nine people tested

	Number of chemicals tested for in all nine people	Total number of chemicals found in people tested	Average number of chemicals found in people tested
PCBs	73	48	33
Dioxins and furans	17	15	14
Organophoshate pesticide metabolites	9	7	3
Organochlorine pesticides and metabolites	23	10	4
Phthalates	6	6	4
Other semi-volatile and volatile chemicals *(24 classes)*	77	77	31
Metals	5	4	2
TOTAL	210	167	91

Source: EWG compilation of blood and urine analysis from two major national laboratories.

The extreme cost of this testing makes it impractical for testing individual patients. Instead, we use Intracellular fluid balance, patient toxic exposure history, and other clinical testing to indirectly assess need for detoxification.

On follow-up Body Composition and Metabolism Assessments (BCM), a decrease of more than .5% of IntraCellular Water (ICW) while losing weight as fat indicates your detoxification pathways are being overloaded. This means we need to further support your detoxification pathways or you will likely go into toxin overload. With toxin overload your metabolism succumbs to poisoning by these toxins and starts to shut down. You then start to gain fat, gain extra fluid to dilute your toxins, and gain weight again.

Successful detoxification is a key issue for sustained fat loss for the many of the patients I work with.

So How Do I Repair My Metabolism?

As Dr. Sid Baker taught me, get rid of the bad stuff and add the good stuff.

For Emma, this is what we found:

1. Emma had low stomach acid and leaky gut problems (see Chapter 2).
2. Emma had IgG and IgA food allergies (delayed food allergies that can create virtually any symptom – or just mess up our metabolism) to the dairy protein found in cow's milk, butter, cheese, yogurt, and ice cream. She also is reacting to wheat and the other gluten containing grains (rye, barley, most oats) and to cane sugar.
3. Emma had medium high levels of lead and mercury on post-chelation challenge toxic heavy metal testing.
4. Emma had real low energy in her acupuncture energy meridians that power her digestion and metabolism. Her body "battery" was run down.
5. Emma's blood laboratory testing showed elevated triglycerides, LDL and total cholesterol, HgA1C, liver enzymes, and hs CRP. These findings indicate poor blood sugar and insulin regulation, excessive inflammation, and a likely fatty liver. Her magnesium, zinc, and iodine levels were low and she was not eating or absorbing enough protein.
6. Emma was eating too many starchy carbs (bread, muffins, pastries, and pasta), too much sugar and sweeteners hidden in processed foods, too much fruit, and too few veggies.
7. Emma wasn't eating enough of the healthy fats that promote fat burning like coconut oil, olive oil, and avocados. Starchy carbs and sweets make us fat – healthy fats make us lean!"

Emma was suffering from insulin resistance. Each time she would consume a slice of bread, a soda, or a sweetened product, her blood sugar and insulin would swing up and down for up to 3 days. This led to "Insulin Resistance" or "Metabolic Syndrome" which means her cell insulin receptor (like a door lock) didn't respond well to her insulin (like a key). Her body made more of the hormone insulin to compensate for this receptor resistance leading to fat gain, increased inflammation, and female hormone imbalances.

This can also trigger elevated cholesterol, triglycerides, polycystic ovarian syndrome, bone loss, and fatty liver.

This is what we recommended:

1. Read labels – if you can't pronounce it, don't eat it.
2. Avoid the white stuff: dairy products, white sugar products, and white flour products. As Dr. Steven Gundry says, "If it's white, keep it out of site!"
3. Eat lots of leafy green veggies and non-starchy veggies of color. "If it is green, it will make you lean!"
4. Go light on the fruit – wild blueberries, organic strawberries, black berries, organic apples are the best of the fruits. Make sure you eat more far more veggies than fruit.
5. Eat at least 5 times per day – 3 protein containing meals and 2 protein containing snacks. Get at least 6 servings per day of concentrated protein (15 gram servings) per day.
6. Get plenty of healthy fats. You heard that right – good fats help our metabolism. Health fats don't make us fat, refined sugars make us fat.
7. Avoid breads, pastas, crackers, cakes, pastries, pies as much as possible.
8. Enjoy legumes in moderation.
9. Keep a food log with someone to encourage and hold you accountable – for Emma it is her Renovare LifeStyle Coach.
10. She met with our Certified Personal trainer who did her strength, fitness, and flexibility assessment and created her aerobic, stretching, and all-important resistance strength program to build muscle. She is meeting with him for exercise training sessions 2X/week for the first 12 weeks to make exercise fun and create healthy habits.
11. Her supplement program was designed to support her metabolism and healthy digestion. This will be revised in 4 weeks after her Body Composition and Metabolism re-testing and again at 8 weeks after her blood laboratory retesting.

12. Her treatment program included microcurrent therapy to help "recharge" her body battery and boost her metabolism. Microcurrent is shown to boost cellular ATP energy production by over 450%. (5)

At the 2 week point Emma reported improved energy, mood, and sleep on her LifeStyle Score. At 4 weeks, she lost 4 pounds of fat, maintained her muscle, and saw a 1% drop in her Intra-Cellular Water (ICW). This means she needed extra detoxification support because burning 4 pounds of body fat released all the toxins stored in this fat – nasties like Dioxin, PCB's, Styrene, and a long list of pesticide and plasticizer residues. This started to overwhelm her liver detoxification ability. We added *DetoxBoost Pro* to her supplement program for this purpose. For Emma, it was crucial that we supported and monitored her detoxification process since the toxic load, if allowed to get too high, would have poisoned her metabolism causing her to gain back fat and weight. (See Chapter 7)

At 8 weeks her blood sugar balance (HgA1C), blood fats (triglycerides and cholesterol), inflammation markers (hs CRP), elevated liver enzymes, low magnesium, and low Vitamin D all showed nice initial improvements.

At 12 weeks, Emma had lost 10 pounds of fat, gained 4 pounds of muscle, lost most of the fluid that made her look bloated and toxic and doubled her energy level. The scale is showing improvement (least important as Emma has learned) and she needs smaller clothes – her waist line is reducing. Her mood, sleep, and enjoyment of life have improved more than she imagined possible. She is getting into the routine of her new LifeStyle and enjoying it.

Family and co-workers are complimenting her and her new friendships that support her on her journey are rewarding, encouraging, and fun. She has a sparkle in her eyes and a spring in her step – she is getting her life back and loving it!

Emma is on track, full of hope, and REALLY encouraged!

Summary:

- If you have failed and failed at dieting, you are not a failure.
- The problem is that diets don't work – they lead to muscle loss and metabolism damage.
- Repairing your metabolism and creating a LifeStyle that fits your unique genetic needs is the only way to long-term success.
- Gaining muscle and metabolic tissue leads to effortless fat loss.
- Instead of dieting, it is essential to "feed" your metabolism so that you gain muscle and boost your metabolism.
- Eating right alone doesn't repair your metabolism – it takes a LifeStyle that fits:
  - Leaky gut repair and digestive wellness
  - Eating smart and removing metabolism-poisoning delayed food allergies
  - Sleep and stress management

- De-stressing and balancing our nervous system
- Supplementing smart
- Exercising smart
- Detoxification of mind and body

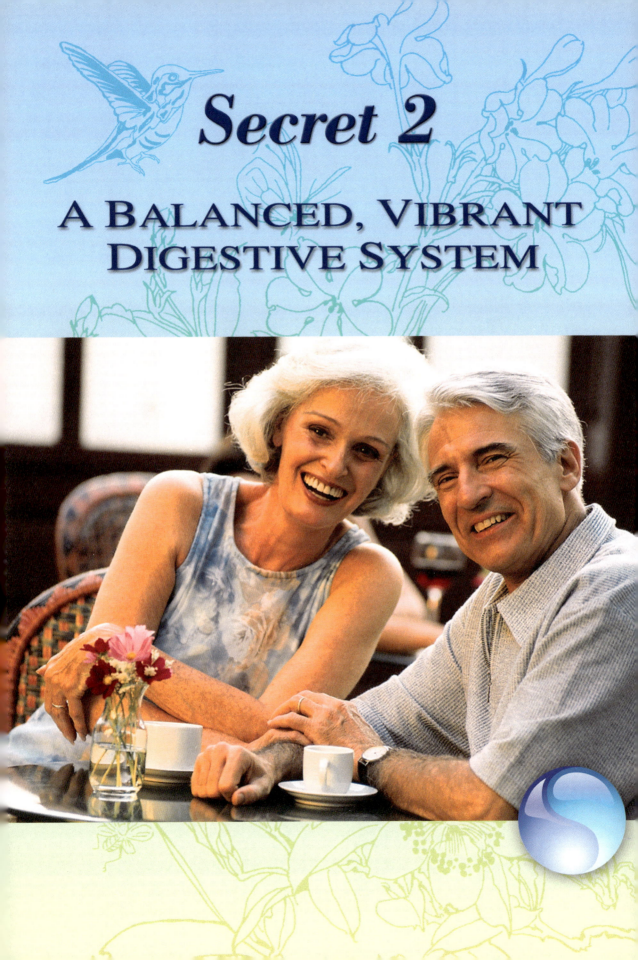

Chapter 2 Snapshot

- Digestive health is the foundation of whole person health – if digestion doesn't work, nothing works well. Without a healthy gut you can't get well or stay well.
- Digestive problems are usually a major "root" or cause of:
  - Fatigue
  - Chronic pain
  - Excessive inflammation
  - Autoimmune disease
  - Blood sugar balance problems
  - Metabolism and weight gain (gaining fat while losing muscle) problems.
- Our Western LifeStyles are especially damaging to our digestive system:
  - Drugs, smoking, excessive alcohol.
  - Excessive stress
  - Lack of sleep
  - Speed eating
  - Junk food
  - Toxins
  - Food allergies
  - Genetically-modified "frankenfoods"
- Leaky Gut (now a recognized medical condition) is becoming more and more common. Antibiotics devastate the tight junctions between the cells that line our gut so they leak like a sieve.
- Food allergies (esp. delayed "stealth" food allergies) appear to affect most of us.
- Gluten and Dairy intolerance or allergy problems are becoming quite prevalent.
- LifeStyle change (rather than popping a pill) is recommended as the "First Line" of therapy/treatment for many digestive problems.
- There is a tried and true approach for repair/healing Leaky Gut– The 4R Program and we have over 25 years experience using it.

There are Two Basic Foundations to Wellness

1. A healthy digestive system with bowel movements 2-3X/day.
2. Deep, restful, rejuvenating, uninterrupted sleep so that you awake feeling recharged and ready to go. We will get to this in Chapter 3.

Without these, you can't get well or stay well. Let's start with the first foundation – <u>Digestive Wellness</u>.

Jennifer's Story

Jennifer was sick and tired of being sick and tired. She had suffered for years with fatigue, chronic pain, gas, bloating, constipation, and emotional mood swings. She slept terribly and had a long list of diagnoses including Irritable Bowel Syndrome, Rheumatoid Arthritis, Fibromyalgia, Premenstrual Syndrome (PMS) and Insomnia. Life was no fun and she was on partial disability. She felt 70 years old yet she had had only 38 birthdays.

Her medical care led to an ever-growing list of medications and her adverse side effects continued to grow as her health continued to slide. As a nurse, she realized that her disease care was not working for her.

When we first met, I just listened with empathy and understanding. What she needed most was someone who cared enough to really listen – this is usually the first step in the healing process.

Then I offered another option for her. I shared the 2004 article from the medical journal "Circulation" describing **"Therapeutic LifeStyle Change"** as the <u>**first step**</u> for many chronic diseases. We talked about going beyond the diagnosis's or labels for her conditions and asking "Why" was her body out of balance and failing to heal.

We talked about her Rheumatoid Arthritis (RA) as one of 180+ autoimmune diseases. I explained that autoimmune disease is simply an immune system out-of-balance – and attacking her joints. I asked her some key questions:

1. Where is your immune system located?
2. What causes your immune system to go out-of-balance?
3. Are there ways to help re-balance your immune system and body overall?

I explained that almost 80% of our immune system is located around our digestive system. Immune cells around our intestines constantly "taste" our gut contents to decide friendly or threatening.

CHAPTER 2 PAGE 19

INTESTINAL HEALTH

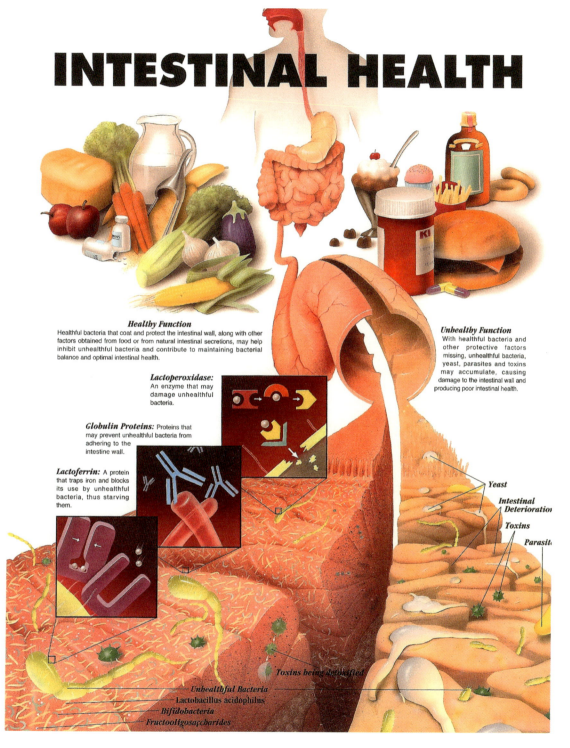

Graphic kindly provided by Metagenics

7 SECRETS TO WELLNESS

The cells that line our gut, as pictured on the left on the previous page, have solid "seals" or tight junctions between cells. These cell junctions provide a protective "inner skin" barrier to leakage. Remember, you have almost 5 POUNDS of microbes living in your gut. Like standing in a septic tank, you don't want your skin to leak!

Antibiotics in particular wreak havoc on these cell junctions – blowing them apart so they leak like a sieve. Junk food, speed eating, food allergies, inadequate stomach acid and toxin overload make things even worse.

Now stuff that is supposed to go into the toilet leaks into our bloodstream. Aggravating things even more, we struggle to absorb the nutrients, vitamins, and minerals from our food and supplements. This hampers our gut repair and can activate our immune system leading to even more inflammation. Leaky Gut causes inflammation and inflammation causes more Leaky Gut – a vicious cycle. Pictured on the right on the previous page is a "leaky gut" with overgrowth of harmful bacteria and intestinal damage. It looks gross and does even worse things to you!

Chronic Inflammation - The "Why" Behind Most Chronic Disease?

I showed Jennifer that chronic (90 days or more in duration) inflammation appears to be the primary "Why" or mechanism behind a long list of chronic diseases:

- Fatigue – due to disruption of cellular energy production
- Colitis
- Crohns's Disease
- Fibromyaglia
- Gastritis (inflammation of stomach)
- Enteritis (inflammation of small intestine)
- Diverticulitis
- Esophagitis
- Bursitis
- Tendonitis
- Heart Disease
- High Blood Pressure
- Alzheimers
- Parkinson's
- Autoimmune Disease (180+ diseases – including Arthritis, Rheumatoid Arthritis, Scleroderma, Lupus, Sjogren's, Vitiligo, Psoriasis etc.)

So Where Does Chronic Inflammation Start?

Inflammation is an immune system tool to deal with perceived threats – like a bacteria infected sliver in your foot. Most of our immune system (over 70%) is located around our digestive system – our gut. So whenever I see chronic inflammation – in joints, lungs, brain, kidneys or anywhere, I first look to the gut for the source of the problem.

So "Why" Chronic Inflammation?

I explained to Jennifer that in my clinical experience, this is what I suspect as "root" issues or causes for her:

- Repeated exposure to antibiotics as a child for her recurring ear infections and frequent colds. Continued antibiotic use as an adult has made things even worse.
- Maldigestion(not enough stomach acid or digestive enzymes and speed eating) and Malabsorption – I have never worked with someone with arthritis in 28 years that didn't have a gut problem.
- Leaky Gut leading to excessive inflammation – remember that most inflammation is started by our immune system and most of our immune system is around our gut.
- Dysbiosis – overgrowth of bad bacteria, viruses, yeast, and spirochetes in the gut.
- Toxin overload – esp. toxic heavy metals like lead, mercury, and aluminum or the myriad toxic chemicals saturating our processed foods and contaminated water supplies.
- Poor detoxification – leading to toxin overload, fatigue, excessive inflammation and pain.
- Excessive stress adding to inflammation and hindering her detoxification and healing ability.
- Depletion of key antioxidant nutrients, vitamins, and minerals.

Jennifer next asked:

"Can I be helped?"

I answered, "In my experience, almost always – as long as you make the recommended LifeStyle changes and we carefully track your response so we can modify your program to fit your unique needs. Since everyone is genetically unique, one-size-fits-all approaches typically fail.

Your body is just "itching to start healing"! We just need to remove enough of the "bad stuff" and add enough of the "good stuff" to support your remarkable self-healing ability.

Jennifer next asked, "How do I get help?"

I answered, "First, I know what does not work - name it, and blame the name. You have "Rheumatoid Arthritis" and you just have to live with it!"

Neither does looking for the "magic bullet" treatment, drug, or supplement. We are a complex biological system. In my experience there are many roots to the health problems of each patient.

Trying to find one "cure" for each problem is like trying to find one simple "fix" for a troubled teenager struggling with drug abuse and juvenile delinquency. As a wise mentor taught me, "Make it as simple as possible, but no simpler".

One of the major changes I have observed in medical research over the past 6 years is the changed focus from single cause to a *Biological Systems* approach.

I showed Jennifer that our body is like a large spider web filling a room. Pull on any part of the web and the whole web shifts. Make any LifeStyle change and it affects our whole interconnected body and our nervous system, digestive system, immune system, hormonal system, neurotransmitter system etc.

What we are learning is that our complex biologic "web" has "nodes" of critical importance. Digestion is one of these. If digestion doesn't work right, nothing works at high level Wellness – especially over time.

I shared with Jennifer that the "4 R" Program for Leaky Gut repair is unusually effective in my 25 years using it since being trained in this by Dr. Jeffrey Bland.

What is the "4 R" Program?

4. **Remove** the bad stuff:
    a. Remove allergic/reactive foods – blood testing of IgG, IgA, and sometimes IgE levels with Blood Food Allergy testing is especially helpful. Skin scratch testing of little value for food allergy testing. Food allergies are almost always an issue —esp. dairy and often gluten allergies.
    b. Suppress excessive overgrowth of harmful yeast, bacteria, and viruses in the gut if needed.
    c. Start a safe, effective, natural parasite removal program if needed.
5. **Replace** the needed Good Stuff:
    a. Stomach acid – as we get older or become fatigued or sick, we make less and less. Nothing works without enough stomach acid to break down and enable absorption of our protein, minerals, and vitamins. Stomach acid also cleans our food of dirty bacteria, yeast, and viruses. Lastly, stomach acid is needed to

signal the valve at the top of our stomach to close properly (think heartburn and GERD), and trigger the release of our pancreatic digestive enzymes.

  b. Digestive enzymes - if needed after correcting stomach acid deficiencies. Important to use pH-independent digestive enzymes if low stomach acid is a problem.

6. **Repair**
  a. L-glutamine, herbs, aloe extracts, and laser acupuncture all seem quite helpful to support repair. Supplying sufficient protein that is adequately digested to amino acids is also important to power the repair process.

7. **Re-inoculate**

I explained to Jennifer that almost 5 lbs. of bacteria live in our gut. When healthy, we have mostly good bacteria and few harmful bacteria. Like a healthy lawn, our good bacteria choke out weeds. To "reseed" a damaged gut we use:

  a. Prebiotics – like fertilizer, promotes growth of healthy bacteria.
  b. Probiotics – like grass seed, promote growth of healthy bacteria. Since we have trillions of bacteria in our gut, high potency probiotics that re-colonize the gut are important. Many brands are 2-4 billion actives per capsule. We now have professional grade probiotics at 100 billion per capsule which are especially effective in practice. To learn more, see the "So Why Different Probiotics?" section in Chapter 5.

So How Do You Know If You Have Gut Problems?

The obvious is pain like:
- Stomach aches
- Gastritis, ulcers
- GERD or heartburn
- Irritable Bowel Syndrome
- Inflammatory Bowel Disease
- Crohn's disease
- Ulcerative Colitis
- Diverticulitis
- Diverticulosis

For some, it's symptoms like:
- Gas
- Bloating
- Constipation
- Diarrhea
- Food intolerance, food allergy, food reactions

For many, they have no gut-related symptoms at all!

A classic example was a jumbo-jet pilot with the classic fighter pilot type A personality. He ran 4-6 miles per day and downed a large bowl of oatmeal every morning for his carbs to fuel his run. He was really health conscious and hated the fact that he needed powerful (and dangerous) corticosteroid inhalers daily to manage his severe asthma. He claimed to have a "cast-iron" stomach – "I can eat anything!"

What do you think I found when we did his exam? After relaxing on his back and bending his knees to relax his stomach muscles, I palpated (pushed in to feel his organs with my fingers). His stomach, small intestine, and large intestine were all exquisitely tender to my palpation– enough that he arched off the table with pain. He was shocked – he had no idea!

Since the gut and lungs develop from the same tissue type in embryology, they are strongly linked. We suspected his asthma was linked in a big way to his gut problems.

After food allergy testing and helping this pilot with the 4R Program, his asthma improved so much that he is free of his need for his corticosteroid inhaler - and he is delighted!

So How Long Does It Take To Repair My Leaky Gut?

Great question! The short answer is I don't know for these reasons:
- Everyone is genetically unique – some heal faster than others.
- If you change your LifeStyle faster, you can expect a faster healing response.
    - Are you getting lots of sleep?
    - Are you relaxing when eating?
    - Are you managing your stress level?
    - Are you consistently taking your recommended supplements?
    - Are you eating lots of the "fresh stuff" that promotes healing.
    - Are you benefiting from treatment to support your gut healing like laser acupuncture and spinal adjusting?
    - Are you taking professional grade supplements that fit your needs to support and accelerate your healing process?
- Consuming your reactive/allergic foods creates a Leaky Gut flare which can take 3 weeks or more to repair. Will you choose to do few or lots of food "experiments" during your healing journey?
- Are you taking drugs that damage the gut and slow healing?

For most, Leaky Gut Repair takes 3 – 12 months. However, some struggle to heal Leaky Gut for years, especially if they lack needed support and continue to make poor LifeStyle choices.

What Do I Do To Get Started?

First step is testing for 2 reasons:

1. Test to know what treatment makes sense for you.
2. Test to <u>measure</u> what does and does not work for you. Since everyone is different, having a measuring tool to evaluate progress (or lack of) is essential. Also, lets us know if you are on the right track even if you don't **yet** feel better.

First, understand that what we do is both a science and an art. Since we could never do enough testing to understand your complex system, we always are guessing. That's why we call it "practice". When we do more testing, we do less guessing.

***My next question for Jennifer was,
"What level of testing do you desire?***

Since Jennifer was sick and tired of being unwell and had suffered for too many years and suffered with too many Doctors, she chose the comprehensive testing option that fit her budget (I also offered her an intermediate and a brief testing option).

We scheduled her exam and testing and her follow-up visit to go over her results.

So What Happened?

Over the next 8 weeks, in a easy step-by-step process with lots of support, Jennifer learned to Eat Smart (Chapter 4), Supplement Smart (Chapter 5), and Exercise Smart (Chapter 6).

We helped her de-stress and rebalance her nervous system and body energy system with spinal treatments and painless energizing laser acupuncture. We trained her in home care laser acupuncture to help her stay energetic, balanced, and peaceful (Chapter 3).

We taught her the Secrets of Deep, Restful, Rejuvenating Sleep (Chapter 3). We added painless ear acupuncture to interrupt her stress cycle that prevented great sleep and we added the sleep-promoting supplements that fit her needs.

Lastly, we helped her learn healthy relationship boundaries, both with herself and others through a referral to our clinic Life Coach and Emotional Release Therapist. This reduced her stress level to allow her to start healing. We also helped her discover what excited her about life and to get a sense of her purpose in life. This shifted her from feeling trapped to hopeful and excited about life again.

So What Were Her Results?

Remember, she had suffered for years with fatigue, chronic pain, gas, bloating, constipation and emotional mood swings. She slept terribly and had a long list of diagnoses including Irritable

Bowel Syndrome, Rheumatoid Arthritits, Fibromyalgia, Premenstrual Syndrome (PMS) and Insomnia.

On a scale of 0 - 10 with 10 being Ideal, 5 medium, and 0 terrible:

- Her energy level improved (over the first 8 weeks) from level 3 to level 7. She has had lots of improvement and has room to get even better.
- Her ability to live free of chronic hand, shoulder, neck, and back pain went from level 2 to level 6 – a real nice start and still work to do. She was encouraged and I explained that Rome wasn't built in a day. It took years to get sick and will typically take months to get well.
- Her ability to live free of gas, bloating, constipation, and digestive pain went from level 2 to level 9. She can't believe how good her gut feels and loves having consistent daily bowel movements. Sounds funny but we celebrated with her when she started to poop daily!
- Her sleep went from level 1 (terrible) to level 6. Lots better and we still have a ways to go. I recommended further neurotransmitter precursor supplement support.
- Her mood improved from level 1 to level 5. We need to help her further balance her neurotransmitters before we are likely to get the results she desires in this area.
- Her PMS and hormonal problems improved from level 2 to level 5. I explained that her hormonal problems are related to her neurotransmitter balance and sleep issues. We need enough deep, restful sleep for effective detoxification essential for hormonal balance. I explained that supporting balanced sleep, detoxification, and neurotransmitter balance would be priority in Stage 2 of her healing process.
- She had lost almost 6 pounds of body fat, started to gain muscle, lost some of her swelling and was encouraged by the comments of her family and friends telling her, "You look better!" This was really encouraging for her since she was eating lots of satisfying, fresh food and was not dieting and never hungry with her new "_LifeStyle For Life_".

Summary:

- If you are not living with high level energy, vitality, and Wellness, your gut is not working right until proven otherwise.
- You can't get well or stay well without a healthy gut.
- A well-done history and exam along with some lab testing will usually do the job sorting out the roots or reasons behind your gut problems.
- Our Western LifeStyles are especially damaging to our digestive system. It takes a concerted effort to stay gut healthy with our junk food, genetically modified "Frankenstein food", and eating out.

- Leaky Gut (now a recognized medical condition) is becoming more and more common.
- Food allergies (esp. delayed "stealth" food allergies) appear to affect most of us.
- Gluten and Dairy intolerance or allergy are becoming quite prevalent.
- We have had a tried and true approach for repair/healing Leaky Gut– The 4R Program and have over 25 years experience using it.
- Remember, step one to getting your health and Wellness back, is heal your gut!

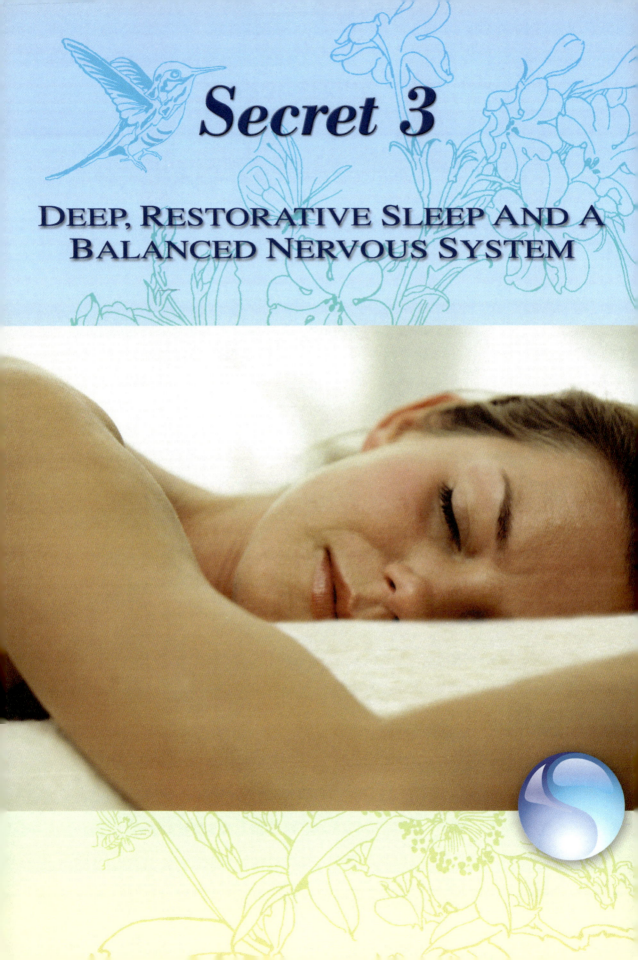

Chapter 3 Snapshot

- Deep, restful, uninterrupted, restorative sleep is a *"**must-have**"* for healing and high-level Wellness.
- Deep healing and repair happen during deep sleep.
- Much of our body detoxification happens during deep sleep.
- Growth hormone which is created during deep sleep has powerful anti-aging effects. Exercise is also great for this – see Chapter 6.
- Deep sleep is a natural anti-inflammatory for our brain and body.
- Deep sleep balances hormones and restores our adrenal glands.
- Deep sleep is needed for neurotransmitter regeneration.
- Deep sleep improves energy, memory, focus, concentration.
- Deep sleep is great for relieving stress – and repairing the effects of stress.
- Sleep problems always have reasons (roots) and uncovering these roots is essential to normalizing sleep effectively, safely, and naturally.
- A balanced, peaceful nervous system is essential to both sleep and high level Wellness.

Janet's Story

Janet desperately needed sleep. She was exhausted and still couldn't sleep – frustrating! When she finally got to sleep, she awoke with the slightest sound or disturbance and struggled – sometime for hours- to get back to sleep. When her morning alarm annoyed her into consciousness, she felt exhausted and ached all over – like she hadn't slept a wink.

Sleeping pills helped only a little, and she felt drugged most of the morning after. Worse, the longer she used them, the less they seemed to help. She knew instinctively that she couldn't go on like this – she must get help.

Janet asked, "What is deep, restorative sleep and how do I know if I am getting it?"

I explained that we must have plenty of stage 4 deep sleep to feel rested, recharged, rejuvenated, and ready–to–roll in the morning. Ideally, we need 7-9 hours of uninterrupted sleep to go through multiple cycles of the stages below:

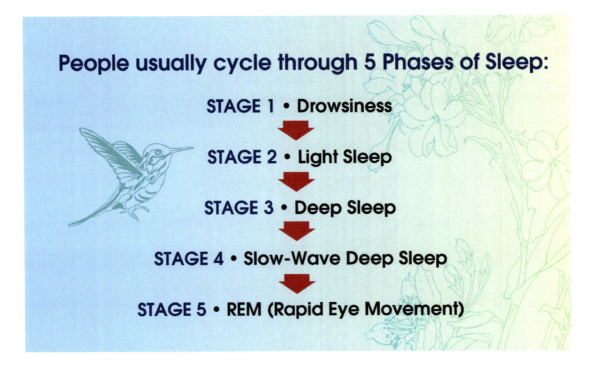

As we delved into her history together, the picture became clearer. Janet had started to have trouble getting to sleep in her early teens. By the time of her college years, it was a real problem. She studied or partied late and slept in late. She tried over the counter sleep drugs and even some prescription sleep drugs with limited success.

At age 24, she has a super-stressful life event – her best friend died of an autoimmune disease. Shortly after, Janet began to develop her digestive problems, fatigue, and chronic muscle and joint pain. Her sleep problems became really bad and she started to hurt all over.

Her downward spiral accelerated and she didn't know where to turn. The long list of prescription drugs no longer seemed to help – instead they seemed to be making things worse. She heard about our safe and effective Renovare natural healing approach and scheduled an appointment with us.

These are some of the reasons (roots) that emerged from her in-depth history:
- Mal-digestion and mal-absorption – she was not absorbing the key vitamins, minerals, and nutrients needed for sleep – especially magnesium to relax her brain,

nerves, and muscles. She also wasn't getting enough protein to provide the amino acid building blocks for the calming neurotransmitters needed for sleep.
- Low Stomach acid – her fatigue, vitamin inadequacy, and high stress compromised her ability to make enough stomach acid to be able to digest her proteins and absorb her minerals properly.
- Food allergies and leaky gut – her food reactions to gluten and dairy were activating her stress response resulting in lots of the stress hormones, cortisol and adrenalin which were keeping her wide-awake at bedtime.
- Poor detoxification and toxin overload – her chemical, heavy metal, and gut bacterial overgrowth toxins were also activating her stress response making sleep even more difficult.
- Blood Sugar and Insulin imbalances – her blood sugar swings were making staying asleep difficult – the low part of the swing (hypoglycemia) would wake her up in the middle of the night.
- Neurotransmitter imbalances – her high stress LifeStyle depleted her calming neurotransmitters and her poor digestion/absorption of proteins – compounded by not enough concentrated protein in her diet – made replacing these sleep-inducing neurotransmitters impossible.

Janet asked, "So What's a Neurotransmitter?"

Great question Janet! Quite simply, neurotransmitters are chemical messengers that allow one nerve cell (neuron) to talk to the next nerve cell.

When we are under lots of stress, we deplete (breakdown) our relaxing neurotransmitters faster than we can make them – especially if we have diet or digestive problems.

These were some of the "roots" we found causing Janet's sleep problems:
- An over-stressed nervous system – her muscle, joint and spinal problems created continuous "noise" in her nervous system – kind of like leaving the bedside clock radio between stations on "static" – with the volume turned up.
- A "Leaky Gut" problem with food allergies was stressing out her "2nd Brain" in her gut. Her gut nervous system was sending stress signals to her brain.
- Neurotransmitter imbalances – especially depletion of her serotonin and GABA reserves were keeping her nervous system in the "go" mode and preventing the relaxed, peaceful, calm needed to promote healthy, deep sleep.
- Blood sugar imbalances messing up her nervous system balance – our brain and nervous system depend on consistent blood sugar balance to work right.
- A bio-energetic or acupuncture system imbalance – her body "battery" was run down and she badly needed a "tune-up".

- A poor sleep environment – her bedroom had light pollution (prevents melatonin production), was too warm, and had too much traffic noise from the street outside. Her mattress and pillow were uncomfortable to make matters even worse.
- Poor sleep habits – she went to bed early, then late, then really late. She had no consistent bedtime to help set her sleep cycle.
- Lack of effective stress management and an imbalanced nervous system
- A pronounced exercise deficiency – see Chapter 6

Janet asked, "Can my insomnia be helped?"

I answered that there is no "cure" for insomnia because everyone is different. Ten people with insomnia each have different sets of "root" reasons. Each insomnia sufferer has a unique LifeStyle and unique genetics. Everyone is different.

What we have found most effective is an individualized approach in which we treat the whole person – not just their insomnia. By identifying the likely "roots" of their problem through your history and testing, we know where to start and how to measure improvement. Since everyone is unique, some of what we will recommend will work for you and some will not. By carefully monitoring and measuring your results, we can "fine-tune" the treatment to best fit your unique needs.

We started Janet on the "4R" program for restoring her gut digestive health (Chapter 2). Since every neurotransmitter needed for sleep in made in our gut as well as our brain, gut health is essential for deep, restful sleep. The "second brain" in our gut is crucial to sleep and nervous system health. This "second brain" in our gut actually has more neurons (nerve cells) than the brain in our skull. Our gut and our brain are intimately linked as shown in diagram on the next page.

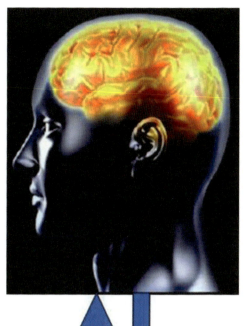

1st Brain

Our Gut—Brain Connection

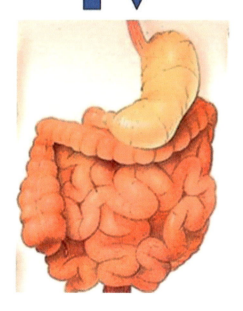

2nd Brain

We also started a program to "de-stress" and "balance" Janet's nervous system.

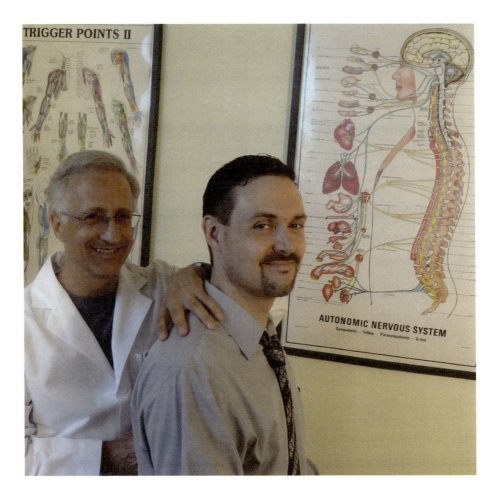

The Autonomic (automatic) Nervous System chart in the background shows how our organs and spinal cord link through our nerves. The picture also shows how we examine spinal function each treatment visit to find the areas of spinal fixation, stress, pain, and inflammation so that we can effectively treat the areas of need. We then re-examine after each visit to ensure that we restored joint movement and function effectively.

For Janet, I explained that our internal stress (inside our body out-of-tune) is often more of a problem than external stress (money problems, mother in law etc.).

Our nervous system receives continuous sensory input from our joints, muscles, tendons, ligaments, and fascia. This sensory input is 200% more than the sensory input from our heart, lungs, liver, kidneys and other organs.

When everything is working just right, this input is like "music" to our brain and nervous system. When our joints are locked up, our muscles are in spasm, and our nerves are over-excitable, this input is "noise" like static on the radio stressing our nervous system from the inside. Imagine living with a radio blasting static at you 24 hours per day – that is STRESS!

Things that help reduce this internal stress and rebalance our nervous system are:

Chiropractic Spinal Adjusting

Each spinal joint level has 7 different directions of movement or "joint play". This is important for the many nerve sensors around each joint to send signals needed for your balance, coordination, muscle control, and nerves to work properly. For some, a gentle and safe Impulse Adjusting Instrument works best to help.

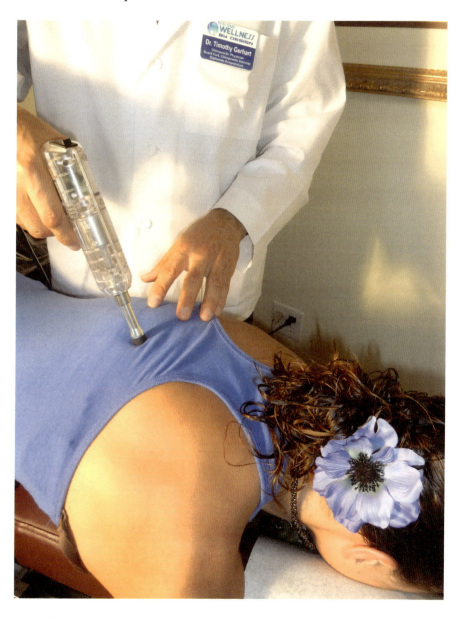

For many, comfortable, hands-on spinal adjusting to help de-stress our nervous system along with Teishein therapy to open key acupuncture energy meridians along the spine works best. Spinal adjusting is even more important to de-stress your nervous system and open bioelectric microcurrent flow than it is for joint health and pain-free flexibility.

For Janet, I recommended 2 treatment visits per week for the first 4 weeks then 1 treatment visit per week for the next 8 weeks combining spinal adjusting to help de-stress and balance her nervous system with microcurrent auriculotherapy and laser acupuncture to help reset her sleep patterns and balance her bioelectric system. Frequency Specific Microcurrent was also used to relax and balance her brain and nervous system on some of her treatment visits.

I relayed that by using an integrated approach (a whole body approach dealing with all of the "roots" of her problems) I accomplish more with one treatment visit now than I did with 3-4 treatment visits earlier in my practice.

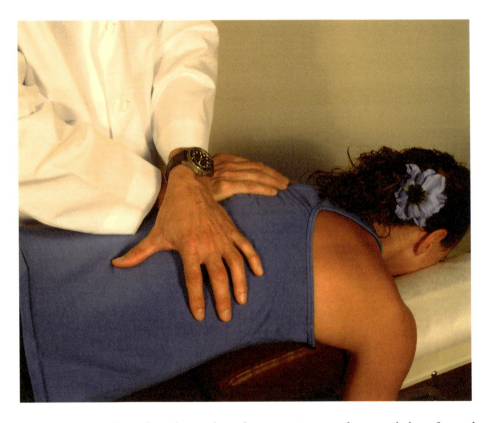

I also let her know that I live this - I have been getting regular spinal, hip, foot, shoulder, wrist, and jaw treatments to correct these joint fixations or locked up areas for the past 30 years to keep my body and nervous system "tuned" like an athlete. I choose this kind of care not only to keep my spinal and other body joints youthful, flexible, and pain-free - I choose this care to keep my nervous system de-stressed, tuned, and balanced to promote my optimal health and Wellness. I look and feel almost half my age as a result.

Acupuncture

Our body has an amazing electrical system like in our homes— but much more complex. We generate electrical current in our body — mostly by our heart contractions. These electrical currents flow throughout our body.

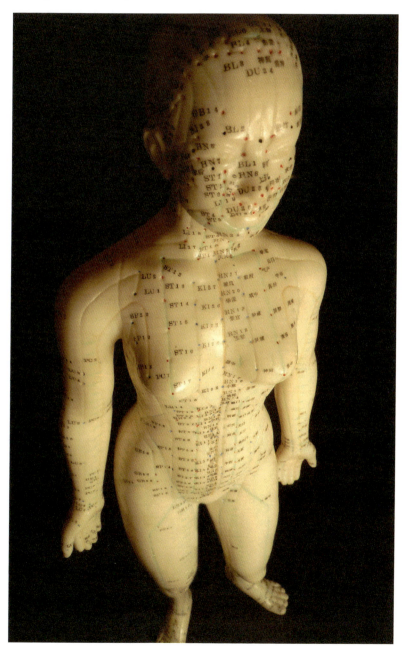

In our homes, we typically have 110 Volts and 15 amps of electrical energy flowing in our wiring. In our body, it is 1.2-1.5 Volts and ultra small amperage in the micro-amp range (one millionth of an amp). These are the same currents measured around the heart with an EKG or around the brain with an ECG.

For most of the un-well people I see, they either have a "low battery" or are way "out of tune" or both. When these electrical currents get blocked, we can experience stress, pain, spasm, or the start of disease.

We use acuheat and laser to recharge patients with a run-down battery and teach them how to treat their "Akabane" points at home with a home laser.

Low level or "cold" lasers are one of my favorite tools to accelerate healing and repair as well as reduce pain and inflammation. We also can do acupuncture with laser for a "needle-free" completely painless treatment approach.

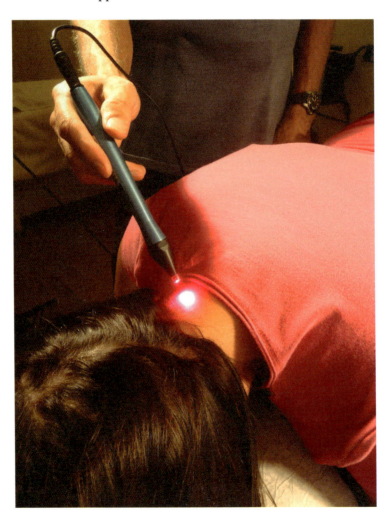

Another laser instrument uses 12 lasers and 12 diodes of various wavelengths in a 3 minute programmed cycles to:

Program 1: Reduce pain and inflammation and energize healing

Program 2: Relax and balance our nervous system

Program 3: Support organ healing and balance

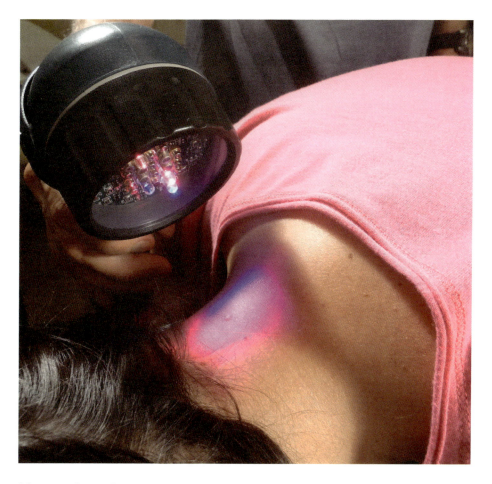

In addition to laser therapy, we use microcurrent therapy to boost cellular ATP energy production. Studies show increased cellular energy production of over 450% with microcurrent therapy.(1) The picture on the next page shows someone receiving soothing microcurrent therapy to her ear points. I love this therapy for me as well!

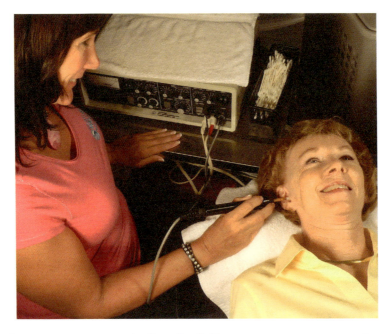

We use foot adjusting to restore pain-free flexibility, treat acupuncture points, and stimulate reflexology points in our feet. When our feet hurt, we seem to hurt all over.

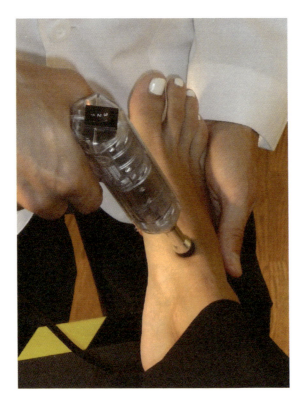

We use acupuncture wires (very thin, usually painless) as well as needle-free acupuncture with healing lasers or microcurrent treatments (very small electrical currents just like your body uses for healing). We sometime use special magnetic patches to treat acupuncture points for an ultra gentle approach.

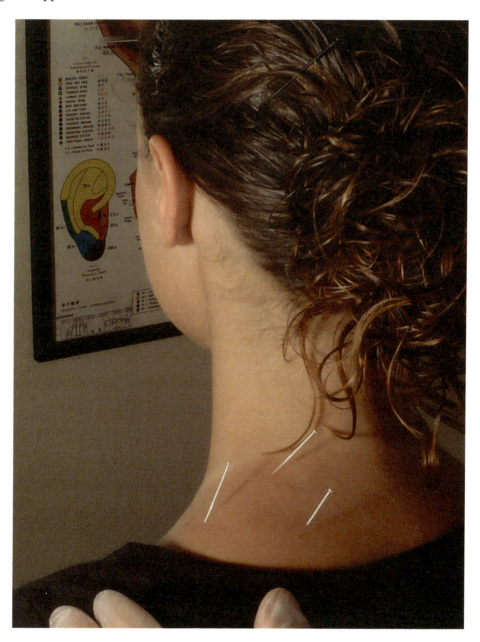

Treating our ear acupuncture points is especially helpful for sleep, mood, and energy problems since the ear points are like the computer keyboard into our brain and central nervous system.

Janet loved her ear point treatments with microcurrent and noticed almost immediate improvements in her sleep and feeling of peacefulness and balance.

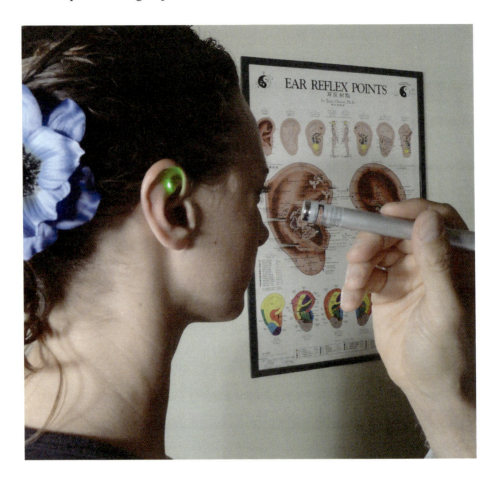

Therapeutic Massage

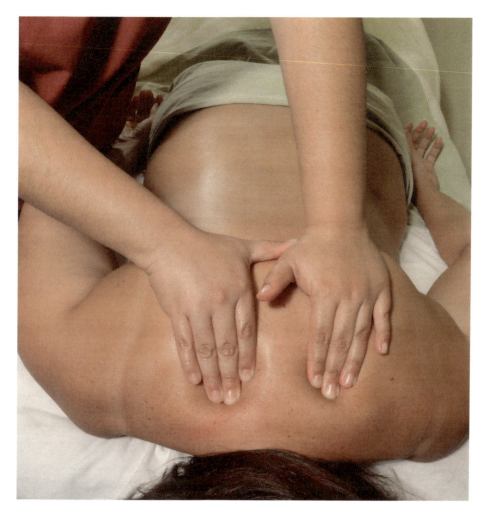

Massage has a long list of potential benefits. For Janet we desired:
- Help relieving stress and relaxation support
- Muscle tension and stiffness relief
- Improved joint flexibility and range of motion
- Deeper and easier breathing through loosening her rib cage
- Decreased mental stress and increased peace of mind
- Increased awareness of her mind-body connection
- Increased feeling of well-being and balance

Janet liked her first therapeutic massage so much that she chose a 2 massage per month package as part of her care program. I relayed to her highly skilled massage therapist the areas of special focus to make her massages most effective.

Janet told me it has been over 2 years since she has taken a real vacation and feels so burdened by caring for everyone else, she doesn't have the time or energy to take care of her.

I asked Janet to remember the last time she flew on a commercial flight. In the pre-flight safety briefing, she was instructed on use of oxygen masks should the cabin de-pressurize during flight. Did they tell you to put the oxygen mask on everyone around you first, and then your own?

Why not?

Obviously, if you don't take care of yourself, how will you be able to care for anyone else?

We talked about this and Janet agreed to the following:
- Schedule 20 minutes for Janet to read, relax, pray, or meditate 6 out of 7 days each week. Janet chose early morning as best so she could combine it with her morning walk to energize her metabolism.
- Schedule a "mini-vacation or extended weekend off" every 8 weeks.
- Schedule a 2 week unwind vacation every 12 months. Going to a quiet retreat center, camping, or a Bed and Breakfast are some of her ideas. Also splurging on an inexpensive 1 week cruise with relax time at home on the front and back end of the cruise.

We also talked about the need to set relational boundaries and learn more about the importance of saying "No" to good things so she could say "Yes" to the best things – like taking care of Janet.

She agreed to make a habit of saying "I need a day to think about it" before automatically saying yes to requests from her church and other social organizations.

I added that we would carefully watch how she responded. If her stress level did not drop as much as desired, we could consider some relaxing herbal based-supplements or targeted amino acid therapy to support her neurotransmitter and nervous system balance.

Janet's Supplement Program

Based on what we learned of Janet's needs, she started on a customized supplement program to support her sleep, relaxation, and nervous system balancing:
- Core 4 Supplements (Chapter 5)
- *MagCitrate Pro* to bowel tolerance (she was able to take (4) 100 mg capules before bed and again first thing in the morning –(5) 100 mg capsules created loose stools so it was beyond her bowel tolerance.
- I LOVE magnesium and virtually every patient needs this since our soil, treated water, and foods are so depleted of magnesium. To make matters even worse, our

stressful lifestyles drain magnesium from our body. Magnesium is vital to help us make peaceful energy and relax our muscles and nerves. If patients develop diarrhea too soon from poor magnesium absorption, we switch to the more highly absorbable Magne*siumGlycinate Pro*.

To get well, Janet MUST sleep well. To help her drop off into deep sleep quickly, along with the magnesium above, I recommended a trusted sleep supporting supplement, *Sleep Perfect Pro Sublingual*. This is great to provide melatonin to protect her brain with its antioxidant effects as well as support her dropping off into deep, restful sleep so she can heal, detoxify, and repair properly. The clinical benefits of *Sleep Perfect Pro Sublingual* are:
- Helps to maintain normal circadian rhythms (our natural, daily sleep/wake hormonal cycles)
- Promotes rapid onset of sleep
- Helps to reset sleep cycles
- Brain anti-oxidant and anti-aging support

Since she had problems with staying asleep, I added my favorite time-released sleep-support supplement, *Sleep Perfect Pro*, to help her stay in deep sleep free of interruptions. Three of each at bed-time worked best initially for Janet. Later, as her system balanced, she did great with just 2 of *Sleep Perfect Sublingual* at bedtime. I like these wonderful brain antioxidant and anti-aging effects so much that I sometimes recommend *Sleep Perfect Pro* for those who don't have sleep problems.

We also helped her to create a "sleep-friendly" LifeStyle by recommending that she:
- Get to bed by 10PM and wake up on a routine schedule
- Turn off her TV, computers, electronics at least a hour before bedtime
- Relax, unwind (read something religious/spiritual, meditate, hot bath) before bedtime
- Avoid allergic/reactive foods
- Consider a high protein snack several hours before bed (high tryptophan foods - turkey, nut butters, figs)
- Avoid grains, sugars, spinach, potatoes, tomatoes, soft cheeses after 7PM
- Avoid caffeine, nicotine, or alcohol at least 6 hours before bedtime
- Avoid exercise at least 2 hours before bedtime. Early morning exercise best
- Reserve her bed for only sleep or sex. She removed the TV from her bedroom and started to read in a chair instead of her bed.
- Keep her bedroom cool but not cold
- Listen to White Noise or wear ear plugs. Relaxation CD's work for some
- Sleep in complete darkness – she started using an eye mask which helped immediately
- Wear socks to bed – cold feet lead to night-time awakening

- Get exposure to bright light in the early morning for her body clock to reset - Janet started 15 minute brisk walks each morning right after awakening

Janet noticed encouraging improvement in her ability to get to sleep, stay asleep, and feel more rested in the morning within the first 7 days of her care program. Not surprisingly, her sleep continues to improve as her overall health and wellness continues to improve. Now she loves her sleep!

Summary:

- We must have deep, restful, uninterrupted, restorative sleep for healing and high-level Wellness.
- Much of our body detoxification happens during deep sleep.
- Anti-aging effects via growth hormone are created during deep sleep.
- Deep Sleep is a natural anti-inflammatory for our brain and body.
- Deep Sleep is needed for neurotransmitter regeneration and body repair.
- Deep Sleep improves our energy, memory, focus, concentration.
- Deep Sleep is great for relieving stress – and repairing the effects of stress.
- We can't feel good and enjoy quality of life without enough deep sleep.
- Sleep problems always have reasons (roots) and uncovering these roots is essential to normalizing sleep effectively, safely, and naturally.
- De-stressing, recharging, and balancing our nervous system is essential for many to regain Wellness

Secret 4

Eating Smart

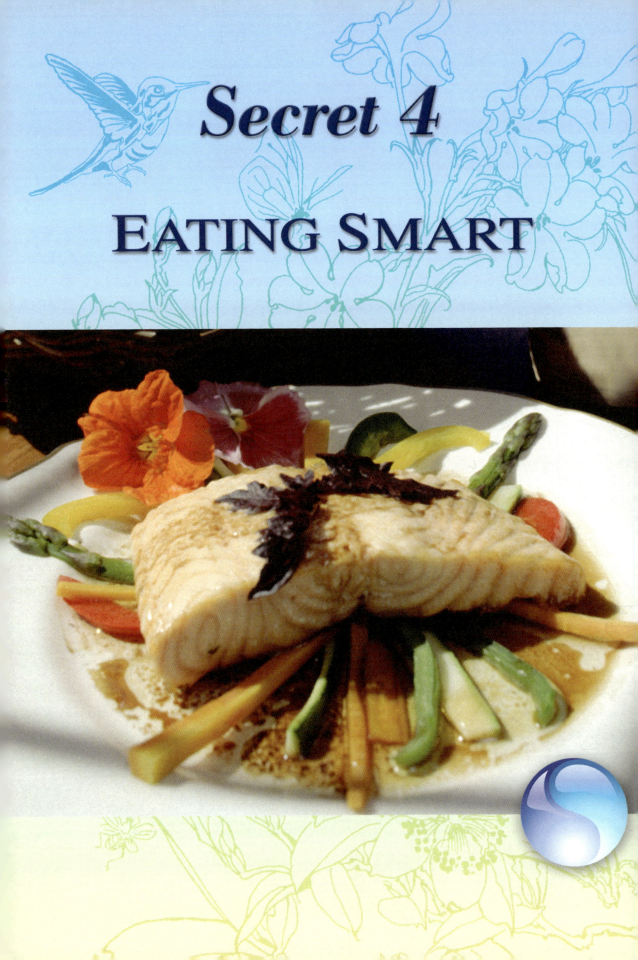

Chapter 4 Snapshot

- We speak to our genetics when we eat.
- Food is much more than just calories – Food is INFORMATION!
- Our eating choices are often the most impactful of our LifeStyle choices.
- Failing to plan is planning to fail
- Delayed Food Allergies are a major problem for most with chronic disease.

Why Eat Smart?

- *Increase Efficient Cellular Energy Production*
- *Increase Stamina*
- *Fight Fatigue*
- *Improve Detoxification*
- *Promote Muscle Gain, Fat Loss*
- *Slow Down Biological Aging*

Here is What You Need to Know

- Everybody is genetically different and what we eat must fit our unique needs for optimum health.
- Some are fast oxidizer metabolic types and need:
  - Lots of concentrated protein – grass-fed beef, organic poultry, fish
  - Plenty of healthy fats
  - Lots of veggies
  - Fewer whole grain carbs

They often consume more calories (of the right type) and larger meals than others and stay lean and fit.

- Some are slow oxidizer metabolic types and need:
  - Less concentrated protein, more legumes (lentils, beans etc.)
  - Less of the healthy fats
  - Lots of veggies, less fruit
  - Some (but not too much) whole grain carbs

They often need fewer calories (of the right types) and smaller meals and find it a bit harder to stay lean and fit. They especially need plenty of exercise and an active lifestyle to stay well.

Most of us are a blend, usually leaning more to one side than the other. What we all have in common is:

- Minimizing refined sugars is really important. The average American now consumes more than 150 POUNDS of refined sweeteners (sugar, high-fructose corn syrup etc.) including an average of almost 50 GALLONS of soda which creates a metabolic and health disaster!
- Most people consume far too many refined carbs (pastries, bread, pasta, cakes, pies, cookies, candy).
- Most of us consume far too little of the fresh stuff of color – esp. fresh veggies. We tend to eat too much fruit and too few veggies.
- Most don't eat often enough and commit the nutritional "Sin" of skipping meals. This stresses our neuro-hormonal system and contributes to blood sugar swings, oxidative stress, adrenal burnout, muscle loss, and fat gain.

We Eat Backwards

Sally is our favorite Bed and Breakfast host in London. She is a delightful host and friend and shared with us what she had learned during her training in a culinary arts school in London. I can hear Sally, in her lovely British accent, saying:

"Feast like a King for breakfast"

"Dine like a Prince for lunch"

"Starve like a Pauper for dinner"

Breakfast needs to be our largest meal. Lunch needs to be our mid-sized meal and dinner needs to be our smallest meal. We tend to do the opposite, leading to increased obesity and even elevated heart attack risk.

Your Vitamin, Mineral, and Nutrient Needs Vary Greatly

- The Recommended Daily Intake (RDI) doesn't apply to you, only to a statistical average person – you are not average!
- The RDI are the minimum (plus a bit) to avoid deficiency diseases in a large population.
- Optimum Health and Wellness needs are usually much higher than the bare minimum RDI.
- Many factors increase your needs greatly.

What Increases Our Need for Vitamins, Minerals, and Nutrients?

- Maldigestion and malabsorption
- Leaky Gut and dysbiosis (overgrowth of harmful bacteria in your gut)
- Low stomach acid
- Food Allergies – especially IgG and IgA delayed types
- Sickness or diseases – from Diabetes to Arthritis to Cancer
- Surgeries, stomach bypass, bowel resections etc.
- Many drugs and medications
- Excessive stress
- Aging
- Lack of sufficient deep, restful, uninterrupted sleep
- Exercise deficiency or excess
- Obesity
- Dieting
- Speed eating
- Constipation or diarrhea
- Damaged metabolism
- Excessive inflammation
- Fatigue
- Too much restaurant food or eating out
- Junk food consumption – excess sugar, rancid fats, and calorie rich, nutrient poor "junk"
- Rancid, contaminated, or inappropriate nutritional supplements – those that do not fit your unique needs
- Poor detoxification and toxin overload

Toxins That Increase Our Nutrient Needs

- Persistent Organic Pollutants (POPs) like DDT, Styrene, Dioxins, PCB's
- Heavy Metals like Lead, Mercury, Cadmium, Aluminum, and Arsenic
- Food preservatives and additives and artificial dyes, colorings
- Excitotoxins like aspartame (NutraSweet), MSG, and flavor enhancers common in processed and restaurant food.
- Artificial Sweetners like Sucralose(Splenda), Saccharin(Sweet and Lo)

Our Food is often Deficient

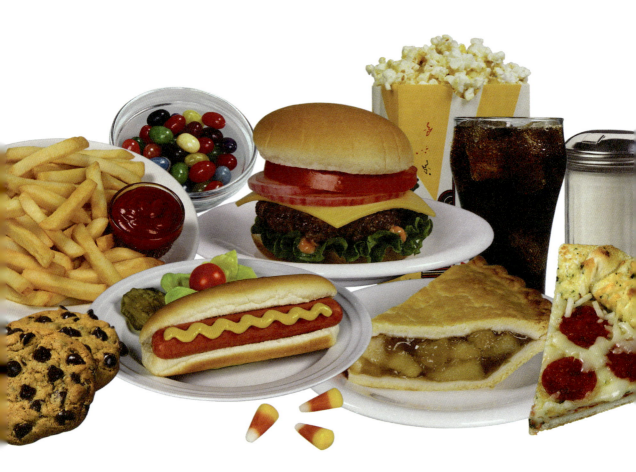

Factory-farmed food has fewer minerals, vitamins than it used to. Our soils are depleted and fertilizers replace only a few of the key nutrients.

Most of our food is no longer fresh leading to loss of vitamin and enzyme activity. Being transported long distances, stored in warehouses, stored on grocery store shelves, and stored in our refrigerator before finally being eaten robs us of much. Fresh is best – buying locally grown produce or growing it in your own garden is ideal.

Most of our food is non-organic. Organic foods are richer in vitamins and minerals and much lower in toxic pesticide and herbicide contamination.

What Do I Eat?

This is the most common question I am asked after sorting through a patient's health history, test results, and LifeStyle treatment plan. Typically, we eat our way to disease and sickness, and we must make some changes if we expect to get well. Doing the same thing and expecting different results in one definition of insanity.

I never fully appreciated the profound impact of our food choices until Dr. Jeffrey Bland, the father of Functional Medicine, explained to me that *food is primarily INFORMATION*. We speak to our genes - our genetics - when we eat. We now know that our genes are like light switches – we turn them on or off with our LifeStyle choices – especially our food choices. The picture below sums it up:

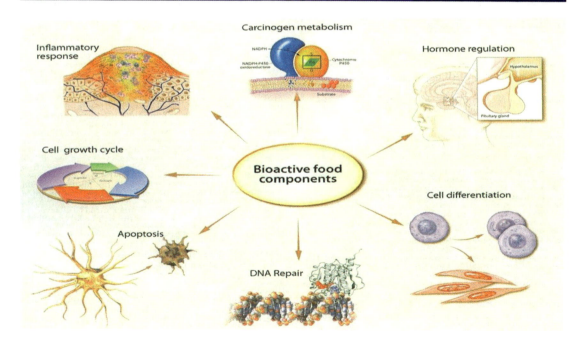

Graphic kindly provided by Metagenics

Our Food Is Information So Our Choices Can

- Turn on genes creating inflammation and dysfunction to increase:
  - Arthritis, asthma
  - Bursitis, tendinitis, myofascitis
  - Degenerative joint and disc disease
  - Chronic pain, migraines
  - Heart disease
  - Alzheimer's dementia, Parkinson's and a long list of brain and nervous system degenerative diseases.
  - Osteopenia, osteoporosis, and muscle loss(sarcopenia)
  - Colitis, gastritis, enteritis
- Turn on genes promoting fibroids and tumors:
  - Uterine fibroids
  - Cancers of many types
- Diabetes, Insulin Resistance
- Obesity and fat gain
- Fatigue
- Depression
- Anxiety
- Brain Fog and poor cognitive function (poor memory, focus, and concentration)
- Accelerated aging

***The less our food has been doctored (processed)
the less we need a doctor.***

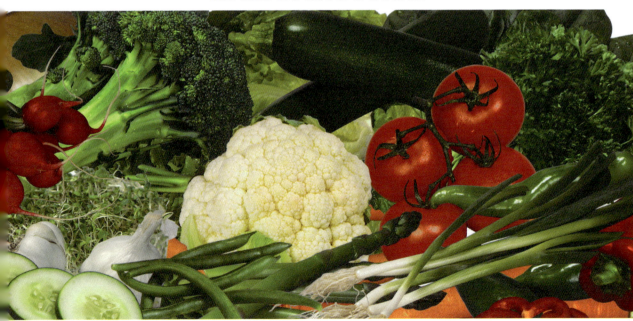

So what's the Good News?

Eating choices that fit our unique needs can also turn off genes promoting disease and inflammation and instead turn on health promoting genes. Our body has a phenomenal ability to repair and rejuvenate. In fact, we turnover everything from our muscles to our bones and get a new body about every 7 years (with exception of most of our brain neurons and some immune blood cell lymphocytes). In a very real sense, we choose our level of health and wellness by our LifeStyle choices. Of these, our food choices are usually the most important.

What if I have made really poor LifeStyle choices and I am a wreck? Is it too late?

I am continually surprised by our phenomenal, sometimes miraculous self-healing ability. This was brought home by our recent "Greatest Loser" contest – a 4 month contest to see who could repair and boost their Metabolism, lose fat, and gain muscle. We had people of all ages enter and participate.

Guess who won?

Surprise! An 82 year old retired nurse who started with serious damaged metabolism and toxicity problems. If she can heal, repair, and boost her metabolism so she looks and feels great, most anyone can.

So How Do I Start?

Step1: Read labels:
- If you can't pronounce it, don't eat it.
- If your Grandmother would not understand the ingredient, don't eat it.
- Avoid Genetically Modified "FrankensteinFoods"(GMO's) Since the powerful food processing corporations have blocked efforts to label GMO foods, buying organic is the best way to avoid these toxic, dangerous foods. USDA organic labeling law does not allow the presence of GMO ingredients.
- The shorter the label the better.
- Best foods have no labels – they are fresh produce.

Step 2: Avoid the "White Stuff":
- "White" (and all other colors of sugar) sugar containing products
- "White" flour (anything not whole grain)products
- Dairy products: Milk, butter, cheese, yogurt (soy and coconut yogurts are fine)

Step 3: Eat lots of fresh veggies and some fruit. See list in resource guide at end of this book.

Step 4: Eat less of refined carbs like breads, rolls, cakes, cookies, pasta, pastries

Step 5: Make sure you are getting enough concentrated protein. See list in resource guide.

Step 6: Make sure you are getting enough healthy fats. Note: Healthy fats don't make us fat (in moderation) - they promote healthy metabolism. Refined carbs and excess sugar damage our metabolism and make us fat.

Step 7: Make a MEAL Plan. This ensures variety and avoids the "Oh My God, I am exhausted and hungry, what can I eat!" crisis which too often leads to regrettable eating choices.

Meal Planning 101

Failing to Plan = Planning to Fail

1. Recipe for failure:
   - When hungry and tired, what do I eat = disaster - especially when only junk available
   - Pantry and fridge stocked with junk
   - Bottom of priority list is food prep and planning

2. Recipe for success:
   - Know what you are eating each day of your week – with flexibility as desired
   - Lots of variety
   - Easy part of your routine – time planned for meal prep and eating
   - Tastes good, good for you, and you feel great after

Creating a Meal Plan is so easy, fast, and simple you will wonder why you didn't do it sooner! It adds variety, flexibility, and makes meal prep and shopping a breeze.

Simple Steps to Meal Planning

1. Choose a concentrated protein source (see Selecting Protein section below) for Monday breakfast, lunch, and dinner.
2. Choose a mid-morning and mid-afternoon snack than also contains protein.
3. Repeat for Tuesday through Thursday.

4. Next, choose a low-starch vegetable for Monday breakfast, lunch, and dinner. (See resource list at end of book)
5. Repeat for Tuesday through Thursday
6. Next, choose a whole grain or starchy vegetable source if desired (See resource list). If repairing metabolism and maximizing fat burning desired, minimize or avoid grains and starchy vegetables
7. Repeat Monday meal plan on Friday, Tuesday meal plan on Saturday, and Wednesday meal plan on Sunday to complete your 7 Day Meal Plan

Helpful Insights

- Breakfast as your largest meal, lunch medium, and dinner small best for metabolism repair and fat loss.
- Breakfast can look like your lunch. If time for breakfast meal prep is difficult, try a breakfast smoothie or shake using one of the recommended functional food powders to supply your protein and nutrients for metabolism boosting. Ask your LifeStyle coach for recommendations.
- How we prepare our foods is also important. Avoid frying, grilling, and scrambling whenever possible. For eggs, poaching, soft or hard boiling best - NEVER scramble as it oxidizes the cholesterol in the eggs. Best for meats is slow temperature cooking: crock pot, simmering on stove top with a stainless steel or ceramic pan containing water. Don't ever use non-stick Teflon type cookware – toxic!!!
- Avoid microwave use whenever possible. Microwaving creates food changes that are quite harmful. Even microwaving water changes molecular structure to create harmful effects to your body and health.
- Remember, a journey starts with a single step. No need to change everything at once or be perfect. Just one small improvement per day adds up to a life-transforming and life-saving LifeStyle in a few short months. *It's about progress, not perfection.*
- Avoid non-stick cookware (highly toxic) and aluminum cookware. Stainless Steel or Ceramic Best.

Creating Your 7 Day Meal Plan

Step 1: Plan your Protein first

How much Protein?
- Your TLC-trained Physician or LifeStyle Coach can use a Body Composition and Metabolism Assessment to measure your metabolism and muscle mass and calculate the amount you need. The minimum for almost everyone is (4) 15 grams servings per day. (6) or more 15 gram protein servings per day is typical.

- Better to be a bit high than too low. Need extra protein to build muscle, power detoxification pathways, regenerate neurotransmitters depleted by stress, and supply cellular repair.

Step 2: Spread protein intake **over 3 meals** and 2 snacks
- (2) 15 gram servings for breakfast
- (2) 15 gram servings for lunch
- (1) 15 gram serving for dinner

Step 3: Spread protein intake **over 2 snacks**
- Ultrameal soy bar - 17 grams of protein
- Ultrameal rice bar - 12 grams of protein
- Complete Boost Pro – 21 grams per 2 scoop serving - great as a shake
- Lean Boost Pro Rice – 15 grams per 2 scoop serving
- Organic apple slices with almond butter
- Veggie slices with organic peanut butter

Step 4: Pick a different protein for each of first 4 days
- Lean meat: grass-fed or organic best 2oz. serving = 15 grams of protein
- Chicken, Turkey: free range/organic best 2oz. serving = 15 grams of protein
- Cold water fish: Salmon, mackerel, trout – Alaskan wild-caught best. 3 oz. serving = 15 grams of protein
- Organic Eggs – 2 large eggs = 15 grams of protein
- Soy/Legumes: beans, tofu, lentils 6oz. serving = 15 grams of protein
- Complete Boost Pro – 1.5 scoop serving = 15 grams of protein
- Lean Boost Pro – 2 scoop serving = 15 grams of protein
- Ultrameal bar – 1 bar = 15 grams of protein

Here is an Example

- Free range chicken on Monday
- Grass-fed beef or organic beef on Tuesday
- Sea-food on Wednesday
- Organic Turkey or Antibiotic-free pork on Thursday
- Free range chicken again on Friday
- Grass-fed beef on Saturday
- Organic Turkey or Antibiotic-free pork again on Sunday

Let's Start filling in your 7 Day Meal Plan. Notice you only create 4 daily meal plans and repeat 3 days to complete your 7 Day plan.

Use the 7 Day Meal Plan in the resource section at end of this book as your template or just copy them.

Pick a Protein Snack for Each Day

You need a protein-containing snack for mid-morning and mid-afternoon.

You also need to rotate your snacks for variety and to avoid developing food intolerance/allergy problems. A handful of almonds does NOT make an effective snack – you need more than this.

A high quality protein-containing shake or an Ultrameal meal bar for snacks are most convenient esp. when traveling or at work. Avoid the supermarket-type slim drinks which contain way too much sugar and allergy inducing dairy protein. Most of these are worse than bad from a metabolism and Wellness perspective.

Step 1: Consider using a concentrated protein – eg. some salmon, meat, tofu, nut-butter for the protein part of your snack.

- 2 tablespoons of organic peanut butter = 9 grams of protein
  = 15 grams of fat
- 2 tablespoons of organic almond butter = 7 grams of protein
  = 16 grams of fat
- 2 tablespoons of organic cashew butter = 5 grams of protein
  = 15 grams of fat

Step 2: You can add apple slices, berries, or a veggie along with your protein source.

Step 3: Write in your snacks for each day of your meal plan.

What About My Vegetables?

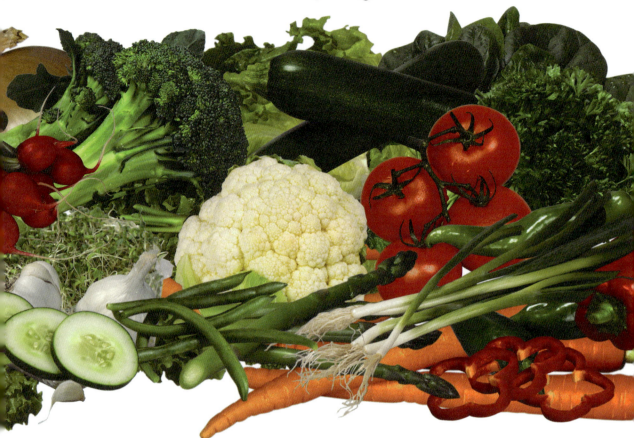

For most of us, we don't get nearly enough veggies. The colors in our veggies have profound health-promoting effects and boost our metabolism. Remember ***"Green makes us Lean!"***

Step 1: Select <u>Non-Starchy Veggies</u> for your meal plan – unlimited amount (minimum of 4 servings per day) See resource list at end of book. Pick a different veggie for Monday through Thursday, can re-use veggie choices for Friday through Sunday

Step 2: <u>Select Starchy Veggies</u> - limit to 1 or fewer servings per day if you desire to repair your metabolism and lose fat while losing weight. See resource list at end of book. Pick a different veggie for Monday through Thursday, can re-use veggie choices for Friday through Sunday

Eat lots of color! When your plate is an artist's palate of color, you are speaking the music of Wellness to your genes!

What about Legumes?

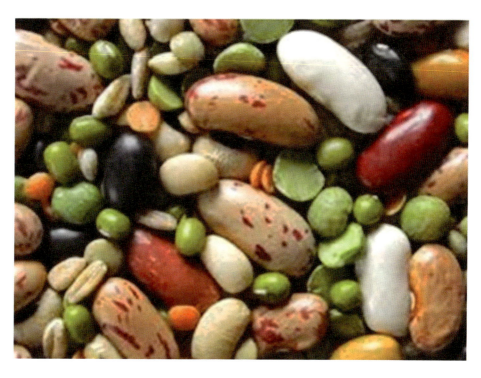

Legumes include peas, peanuts, and many types of beans. They are great sources of protein, fiber, nutrients, and wonderful for supporting balanced blood sugar and metabolic syndrome repair. They are budget-friendly and usually available as organic:
- Adzuki or Aduki or Red Beans
- Black beans
- Black-eyed peas
- Garbanzo beans – also called Chickpeas (used to make hummus)
- Great Northern beans
- Kidney beans
- Lentils – regular and black lentils which are my favorite
- Lima beans
- Mung beans
- Navy beans
- Pinto beans
- Red beans
- Soy beans – use organic only – GMO soybeans have health issues that are serious.
- Split peas

Add legumes as desired to your Meal Plan using the resource guide at end of this book.

Wrapping It Up

Oils: Use healthy oils such as Extra Virgin Olive oil (preferred) or Canola oil for cooking. Other oils recommended are Grape seed oil, Coconut oil, Walnut oil, and Flaxseed oil. Be extra careful with flaxseed oil in that it oxidizes and goes rancid easily. I recommend organic oils packed with nitrogen in the glass bottle to replace oxygen. Always refrigerate.

Fruit: Use fruits from ideal fruit section in Resource guide at end of this book. Remember to eat more veggies than fruit and 2-3 servings per day maximum. A organic apple medium size or ½ cantaloupe is one serving.

Dairy: I recommend dairy free for at least first your first 30 days of Eating Smart. I have seen so many food allergy/intolerance problems over the years that I now assume dairy protein allergy or intolerance until proven otherwise. These reactions can be delayed and trigger everything from arthritis, blood sugar elevations, and sinus problems to fat gain.

Grains: I recommend minimizing your bread, pasta, and cereal grain consumption to promote insulin sensitivity and improved blood sugar balance and fat loss. As you become healthier, most can gradually add small amounts of organic whole grain products. Be careful not to overdo this if you want to stay lean, trim, fit, and healthy.

What do I Drink?

The best option is water purified at point of use. Never drink unfiltered tapwater! The best solution for most is a filter below your kitchen sink with a separate faucet to use for all of your drinking and cooking needs.

The filters that typically come with a fridge remove some of the chlorine to make your water taste better. They do virtually nothing to remove the host of toxic chemicals in our water supply. I use a separate *Multipure* water filter above our refrigerator that purifies the water before it reaches our ice maker and cold water dispenser.

I have recommended *Multipure* water filter systems for over 25 years. It does the best job of removing most of what we don't want in our water, while leaving most of what we do want. It is economical (about 1/10th the cost of bottled water) and certified by the National Sanitation Foundation to remove a long list of "bad stuff".

A high quality Reverse Osmosis (RO) system also does a good job as long as the filters are serviced (replaced) regularly. I personally use a Multipure filter combined with a RO system under our kitchen sink to do the best job filtering out the myriad toxic compounds that pollute our water supply.

Green Tea, White Tea, and a long list of herbal teas are also great, healthy drink options. The tea polyphenols have a long list of health promoting benefits – including metabolism support for fat loss.

Coffee does have health benefits as long as used in moderation and you don't have an allergy or sensitivity. Remember, the delayed allergies are stealth – you don't notice a change after drinking coffee – the immune response can occur hours or even days later and the only symptom may be fat gain.

Always use organic coffee and limit to 2 cups per day max, preferably in the AM. Rotate with herbal teas to minimize development of an allergy to coffee. The other major issue is toxicity – use ONLY ORGANIC coffee – you don't want the pesticide residues with your coffee.

If using juices, organic is best and ALWAYS dilute them at least 50:50 with pure water to avoid spiking your blood sugar. If using pomegranate, cranberry, lemon, or lime juice or something else that needs sweetening, best to use stevia as a sweetener and avoid added sugar and always avoid artificial sweeteners - toxic!

Nature's Sweet Pro is my favorite calorie-free health-promoting sweetener. It is a special variety of Stevia derived from the Morita plant and it is the only Stevia in the world grown organically. It supports farmers in Columbia, South America as they switch from cocaine production and is the smoothest Stevia I have ever tasted – free of the bitter aftertaste of other types of Stevia.

If you desire to add milk to tea or coffee, organic soy, coconut, almond, hemp or hazelnut milks work well. Avoid artificial crème-type products – toxic!

How Do I Eat Out?

Eating out at restaurants and promoting your health do not go together well. Reserving eating out for special events and as an occasional treat is best if you are serious about pursuing Wellness. For when you do eat out:

1. Always have a meal bar with as a backup.
2. Eat first at home if possible.
3. Choose a full menu (sit-down) restaurant or a restaurant from a gluten-free restaurant list.
4. Choose brown rice, not white.
5. Tell waiter you need gluten and dairy free choices and do best you can. Eg. Small amount butter on veggies may be best you can do.
6. Remember, the less you eat out, the healthier you will be.
7. Some of our patients use a surprisingly effective supplement, *Histoblock Pro*, to help reduce their allergy reaction when eating out.

Recipes

1. Choose from your favorite recipes and substitute the protein and veggie selections as desired.

2. I especially like the "Paleo Diet" (see suggested reading in resource guide at end of this book) approach for repairing metabolism for those with insulin resistance and excess fat with too little muscle. The second half of the book is quick and simple recipes.

3. For those (like me) who prefer quick and easy, I do "food assembly" and avoid complicated and time-intensive recipes.

Good, fresh, healthy food tastes good without need to do much to it.

Shopping List creation

1. Try Natural food grocery stores like Sprouts, Whole Foods, Trader Joes and learn the selection of what they stock. Always try one new thing each shopping trip to expand your food horizons – especially a new veggie. Also, visiting a local Farmer's Market is a great way to get super fresh healthy food from the people who grew it. And even the big box stores like Costco now carry organic ground beef.

2. Start a garden! Picking fresh stuff from my garden to eat is always a joy.

3. Keep a shopping list in your kitchen so when you run out of something, it gets restocked.

Stocking Your Pantry and Refrigerator

1. What to throw out – the junk! Review the "White Stuff" list above.

2. What to purchase:

   Condiments: Redmond Sea Salt, Organic Ketchup, Balsamic Vinager, Tasty Mustards, Horseradish are a start. Dairy-free mayonnaise such as Veganaise are great to have on hand. I also REALLY like *Earth Balance* spread as a great tasting alternative to butter for eating and cooking.

   Spices: ginger, garlic, chilli, cinnamon, tumeric, black pepper, oregano, coriander, cumin, fenugreek and mustard are a start to add to taste and health benefits.

   Basics to always have on hand:
   - Organic brown rice cakes
   - Organic Cashew and Almond butter.
   - Honey and an organic fruit spread free of added sugar or sweeteners.
   - A selection of nut and seeds: cashews, walnuts, pecans, pepitas(pumpkin seeds), sunflower seeds.

What about Food Allergies?

<u>Delayed</u> Food Allergies can cause virtually any symptom anywhere in your body. The problems they cause are rarely limited to your digestive system.

Delayed means IgG mediated(IgG immune pathway) = hours up to 3 days after consumption before symptoms manifest. IgA immune pathways are also important for many. Special IgG and IgA blood food allergy panels are used to find these problems. Typical allergists rarely test these pathways.

This is in contrast to IgE mediated = minutes to hours after eating before you notice symptoms. Classical allergies to shellfish, peanuts, and strawberries that can create life-threatening problems are IgE mediated. They can be picked up with scratch testing of your skin and blood IgE testing. This is the testing typically ordered when you ask you medical physician or allergist for "Allergy" testing. Unfortunately, IgE testing misses the vast majority of significant food allergies. There is now evidence of a delayed-type IgE food allergy reaction as well.

Lab testing for allergies is both an art and a science. Because there are many immune pathways and we can only economically test a few, a positive test means you are reactive and must avoid the offending food. A negative test result does not always mean the food is safe for you – your food reaction may be via an immune pathway that we did NOT test. Our standard 96 food panel usually gives us enough info to figure out the puzzle – especially when we carefully watch how you respond to your customized "Eat Smart" program.

<u>Food allergies always have "roots" or causes.</u> The most common:
- Leaky gut which causes partially digested food to leak into your bloodstream triggering an immune "allergy" response.
- Insufficient stomach acid or digestive enzymes creating a barrage of partially digested food particles leaking into your bloodstream.
- Speed eating which causes all kinds of trouble.
- Different medications – esp. prolonged use of acid blockers and antibiotics.
- Disruption of gut microflora and overgrowth of harmful microbes (dysbiosis).
- Emotional Stress Overload – esp. on a subconscious level. Chapter 7 goes into this topic further.

To Clear Food Allergies

- Heal the gut with the "4R" program described in Chapter 2.
- Deal with any other "roots" or causes.
- Help your immune system "unwind" or "calm down" with spinal adjusting, acupuncture, laser therapies, microcurrent therapies, and Frequency Specific Microcurrent (FSM).

- Release our emotional stress on a conscious and a subconscious level. I find Emotional Release Therapy and Guided Mental Relaxation Therapy especially helpful. You can learn more about these therapies in Chapter 7.
- Avoid the offending foods long enough for your immune activation to calm down and return to normal. For some this is 3 months, for others it takes 6 months or longer – esp. if their leaky gut problems are slow to heal because of repeated "experiments" involving eating their reactive foods too soon.
- Avoid food "experiments" damage the gut lining leading to "Leaky Gut" for 3 weeks or longer after each exposure.

Sometimes, the allergy or food intolerance will not go away. This is especially common with Gluten and Dairy. Long-term avoidance is essential to Wellness in these cases.

The Gluten Conundrum

- 30% of Americans have gluten sensitivity
- 81% of Americans have a genetic disposition to gluten sensitivity
- 95% of all processed foods contain some form of gluten.
- Wheat has been bioengineered to boost gluten 90% more than what our grandparents ate.
- No lab test exists that shows that gluten is safe for you.
- Lab testing to show gluten sensitivity is a complex art - easy to miss.
- The average American suffering from severe gluten intolerance (celiac disease) suffers from Doctor to Doctor for 10 years before being diagnosed
- Gluten avoidance is just the start of healing and repair. Identifying ALL of your reactive foods and dealing with gut healing (4R program) and eliminating the causes of your damage gut is essential

So What Is Gluten?

Gluten is a form of protein found in wheat (all types including semolina and durum), spelt, rye, barley, triticale and most oats.

Gluten Intolerance affects almost 30% of our population and can cause virtually any inflammation or autoimmune symptom and is easy to miss and hard to diagnose. Celiac Disease is the extreme of gluten intolerance. You can be gluten intolerant without meeting the medical diagnostic criteria for Celiac Disease. If you Doctor says you don't have Celiac Disease, you may still be intolerant to gluten.

What Symptoms or Diseases are linked to Gluten Intolerance?

- Rheumatoid and "Wear and Tear" Osteoarthritis
- Tourette's Syndrome
- Rosacea, Dermatiformis, Eczema, Psoriasis, and other skin problems.
- Hashimotos's thyroiditis, hypothyroid, and most thyroid problems.
- Multiple Sclerosis (MS), Amyotrophic lateral sclerosis (ALS), Scleroderma, Sjogren's, and other Autoimmune Diseases.
- Weight gain in some and weight loss in others.
- Diabetes and elevated blood sugar.
- Metabolic syndrome with elevated insulin, cholesterol, triglycerides, and blood pressure.
- Depression, Anxiety, Sleep Problems, Brain Fog, Dementia, Schizophrenia, Neuropathies, ADD, ADHD, and Alzheimer's dementia symptoms.
- Non-Alcoholic Fatty Liver Disease (NAFLD) or Fatty Liver which affects 30% of Americans.
- Osteoporosis and Osteopenia (it is now recommended that ALL people suffering with bone loss be tested)
- Colitis, Crohn's, Irritable Bowel Syndrome (IBS), GERD and heartburn.
- Increased Heart Disease and Cancer risk.

Gluten-containing Grains

- Wheat and Barley
- Barley malt/extract, maltodextrin
- Bran
- Bulgur
- Couscous or tabouli
- Durum
- Einkorn
- Farina
- Faro
- Graham flour/crackers
- Kamut
- Matzo flour/meal
- Orzo
- Panko
- Rye

- Seitan
- Semolina
- Spelt
- Triticale
- Udon
- Wheat bran, hydrolyzed wheat protein

Other Foods/Ingredients That May Contain Gluten

- Beer and lagers
- Breading and stuffing
- Brown rice syrup
- Dry soup mixes or soup bases
- Hot dogs
- Meat sauces/tomato sauces
- Monosodium glutamate
- Nondairy creamers
- Some herbal teas and instant coffees
- Sour cream, ice cream, puddings
- Soy sauce or teriyaki sauce (unless labeled gluten-free

The Gluten-containing grains list and the Foods/Ingredients That May Contain Gluten list are from (1)

Avoid Gluten in Disguise

The following list gives words and phrases that could spell danger and are best avoided on a gluten free diet.

- Flavorings unless specified with each being gluten-free
- Edible or Food Starch
- Fillers
- Seasonings
- Binders
- Rusk
- Bran
- Wheat germ
- Wheat protein
- Wholegrain
- Thickening

- Wheat starch
- Malt – this is a major source of gluten hidden in breakfast cereals, beers, and milkshakes. Gluten-free beer is available and tastes great.
- Maltodexrin – usually derived from barley and contains gluten

What Do I Eat That's Gluten-Free?

Lots of things are now available. Virtually anything you eat with gluten is now available gluten-free. You just need to know where to look. Whole Foods Market and Sprouts Farmers Market (1) have a huge number of gluten-free selections. Some of the gluten-free pastas are so good I have Italian pasta connoisseurs choosing gluten-free pasta because it tastes better than the gluten-containing types.

Foods you CAN eat on a gluten-free diet include:
- Rice – use organic brown rice only
- Corn – use only organic to reduce risk of GMO contamination
- Potatoes (yellow flesh or Yukon gold potatoes have the lowest glycemic index)
- Yams
- Sweet Potatoes
- Quinoa (a tasty high-protein grain from the Inca's that you cook just like rice)
- Buckwheat (grain or flour)
- Almonds, Cashews, Pecans, Macedamia nuts, Filberts
- Fruits and Vegetables
- Beans, Peas, Soy milk, Soy Cheese, Tofu
- Fresh meats and fish (unbreaded)
- Arrowroot (great for a gluten-free thickener)
- Tapioca

Eating Smart is one of the most important of our LifeStyle choices. It determines our level of energy, vitality, and Wellness more than almost any other LifeStyle choice. Managing our thoughts, emotions, and stress would be a close second (Chapter 7) and often they are related – think emotional eating.

When people tell me "I am not the planning type" when it comes to food choices, I ask them if they plan for a vacation or trip? Failing to plan is planning to fail. With very few exceptions, those who have a 7 day meal plan are the most successful. Planning actually results in freedom – not stuck in a rut. Your meal plan allows lots of flexibility – you just have a plan to start with and fall back to when needed. Remember to seek out the help and support you need to create your Meal Plan and Eat Smart program.

Summary:
- We speak to our genetics when we eat.
- Food is much more than just calories – Food is INFORMATION!

- Our eating choices are often the most impactful of our LifeStyle choices.
- Food Allergies are a major problem for most with chronic disease.
- Everybody is genetically different and what we eat must fit our unique needs for optimum health.
  - Fast oxidizer type
  - Slow oxidizer type
  - Mixed oxidizer type
- Meal planning takes the stress and hassle out of Eating Smart
- Almost everyone needs support and encouragement on the change journey to Eating Smart.

Secret 5

SUPPLEMENTING SMART

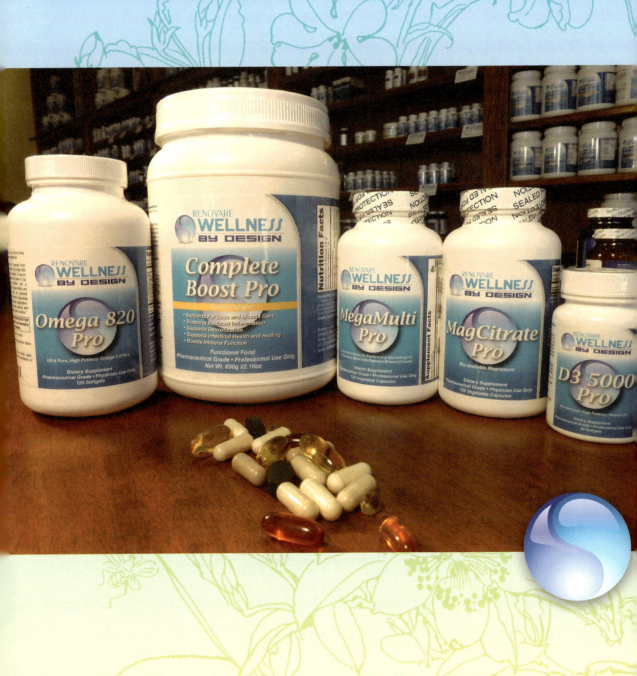

Chapter 5 Snapshot

- Few of us get even the bare minimum or recommended daily intake (RDI) of all of our essential vitamins, minerals, and nutrients.
- Our stressful lifestyles, fast food, gut problems, and toxic load further increase our needs.
- Our pandemic of chronic disease is caused in part by deficiencies or being sub-optimum in these key vitamins, minerals, and nutrients.
- Supplementing Smart is a crucial part of creating a LifeStyle supporting Wellness.
- An ounce of prevention through supplementing smart is worth more than many pounds of cure.
- Everyone is different so our supplement program needs to fit our unique needs – and change as we change.
- Testing is available to assess our needs and monitor our response to our supplement program.
- Supplements are a "supplement" to eating smart and do NOT replace smart eating.

So Why The Need For Supplements?

Our soils and food are depleted of many of our essential Vitamins, Minerals, and Nutrients. Our food choices are often less than ideal and our stressful lifestyles increase our needs far more than our food choices supply. To make matters worse, aging, fatigue, mal-digestion, mal-absorption, medications, and toxicity increase our needs even more. For those suffering with illness or disease, nutrient needs become even greater and more critical.

Americans Are Chronically Malnourished

The **National Health and Nutrition Examination Survey** (NHANES) report, released from the USDA-ARS Food Surveys Research Group (FSRG), finds that too many Americans have inadequate intake of key essential nutrients.

The new report is titled, ***What We Eat in America*** and covers the period of 2001-2002. The data is based on self-reported "24-hour recall" from those participating in the data collection. (1)

What the data tells us is clear - Americans are deficient in key nutrients.

The most alarming shortfalls were found for:
- Vitamin E
- Vitamin C
- Vitamin A
- Selenium
- Magnesium
- Potassium

Other studies have consistently shown Vitamin D deficiency is a problem in the United States.

The reason why it is so important to strive for nutrient adequacy every single day is that falling short of even a few vitamins, minerals or trace elements has a profound impact on your health **because** *all vitamins, minerals and trace elements are intricately dependent on each other in your body.*

To understand how this works, let's look at the nutrients this data suggest Americans are falling short for:

- **Vitamin E** is intricately connected to: Vitamin C, glutathione, selenium, and Vitamin B3.
- **Vitamin C** has significant interactions with several key minerals in the body - it enhances iron uptake and is required for regeneration of Vitamin E. Both Vitamins C & E appear to work together as powerful antioxidants and in the survey *both were found to be deficient.*
- **Vitamin A requires** adequate intake of dietary fat and zinc which are necessary for the absorption and utilization of Vitamin A.
- **Selenium** is indirectly responsible for keeping the body's supply of at least three other nutrients intact - Vitamin C, glutathione, and Vitamin E. The chemistry of these relationships is complicated and centers around an enzyme called glutathione peroxidase. Glutathione is central to both toxic chemical and heavy metal detoxification.
- **Magnesium** is required for cell membrane stability, making energy, and keeping your muscles and nerves relaxed and balanced. (*More on this in Core 4 Magnesium section*)
- **Potassium** works in the body through a mechanism known as the "sodium-potassium" pump - sodium and potassium work together to initiate muscle contraction and nerve transmission, and to maintain the body's normal distribution of fluid. Adequate intake of potassium is as important as adequate intake of Vitamin D and magnesium for bone health.

- **Vitamin D** plays a major role in maintaining normal blood levels of calcium and impacts the absorption and storage of calcium. Vitamin D also helps to control over 2000 genes that impact our immune system and inflammation. Vitamin D also regulates the production of certain calcium-binding proteins that function in the bones and kidneys. Because these binding proteins are dependent on Vitamin K, there is an interrelationship between Vitamin D and Vitamin K. Vitamin D deficiency may also result in iron deficiency. (*More on this in Core 4 Vitamin D section and the Vitamin K section*)

So, while some levels of nutrients were found to meet the bare minimum RDI levels, very real deficiencies were noted. This means that even when some nutrients meet RDI levels, the shortfall of the deficient nutrients impacts the bioavailability of the RDI adequate nutrients. This is why it is so important to strive for nutrient adequacy every single day.

So What Do I Need For My Optimum Health?

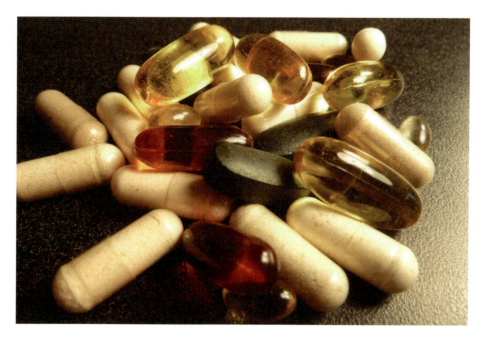

Bruce Ames, professor of Biochemistry and Molecular Biology at the University of California, Berkeley, and a senior scientist at Children's Hospital Oakland Research Institute (CHORI), suggests that "to maximize human health and lifespan, scientists must abandon outdated models of micronutrients" and that "a metabolic tune-up through an improved supply of micronutrients is likely to have great health benefits. (2)

In my past 25 years of practice involving blood laboratory testing and nutritional evaluations, virtually everyone needs the "*Core 4*":

Core1: ***Mega Multi Pro*** - Professional-grade Multiple Vitamin/Mineral.

Core2: ***Omega 820 Pro*** – Contaminant and rancid-free highest potency on the market Omega 3 EPA-DHA fish oil concentrate.

Core3: ***D-3 5000 Pro*** – almost everyone tests suboptimum on Vitamin D-3 which is a critical regulator of cell energy and health.

Core4: ***Magnesium Citrate Pro*** -essential for energy, metabolism, weight management, heart health, and staying well.

Why Do We Need A Multiple Vitamin/Mineral?

In 2002, a paper by Robert H. Fletcher and Kathleen M. Fairfield from the Harvard School of Medicine, published in the Journal of the American Medical Association, they state that "it appears prudent for all adults to take vitamin supplements." In this article, which examined the clinical applications of vitamins for the prevention of chronic diseases in adults, they examined English-language articles about vitamins in relation to chronic diseases published between 1966 and 2002, and concluded that inadequate intake of several vitamins has been linked to the development of diseases including coronary heart disease, cancer, and osteoporosis. (3)

Similarly, the April 9, 1998 issue of the New England Journal of Medicine featured an editorial entitled "Eat Right and Take a Multivitamin" that was based on studies that showed health benefits resulting from the consumption of supplemental folate to prevent birth defects and possibly decrease the incidence of cardiovascular disease. (4)

So Which Multiple Vitamin/Mineral Do I Need?

In my years of clinical practice, I have found that virtually everyone needs more than they can get in a one-a-day multiple Vitamin/Mineral. Our poor diets, soil nutrient depletion, mal-digestion, mal-absorption, medications, toxicity, disease, and excessive stress are just a few of the reasons for increased supplemental needs. You just can't fit what you need into one tablet or capsule and still be able to swallow it.

To get the job done, a professional grade 4/day Multiple Vitamin/Mineral designed to be taken as 2/meal, 2X/day is the least for most people I have evaluated through nutritional assessments and lab testing. For others, a 6/day or 8/day Multiple is needed to meet their needs. One of my favorites, Mega Multi Pro, is surprisingly affordable and effective at 4 to 6/day.

Core1: ***Mega Multi Pro*** - Professional-grade Multiple Vitamin/mineral that supports:
- Insulin sensitivity for fat loss and muscle gain
- Cellular energy production
- Antioxidant protective support
- Reduced pain and inflammation
- Reduced cardiovascular risk

- Balanced blood pressure
- Healthy brain and heart function
- Protection of our vision and kidneys
- Decreased disease risk
- Strong, balanced immune system function
- Detoxification and anti-aging

Core2: ***Omega 820 Pro*** – Contaminant and rancid-free highest potency on the market non-prescription Omega 3 fish oil concentrate that supports:
- Reduced pain and inflammation
- Reduced cardiovascular risk
- Balanced blood pressure
- Balanced HDL/LDL cholesterol and triglycerides
- Anti-diabetic and anti-oxidant effects
- Prevention and management of arthritis & other autoimmune diseases
- Weight loss through muscle gain and fat loss
- Healthy brain development during pregnancy
- Protection of our vision and kidneys
- Decreased Alzheimer's risk
- Immune system health and balance
- Skin health:
  - Reduced wrinkling.
  - Slowing of unhealthy aging of our skin.
  - Reduced dryness.
  - Reduced skin cancer risk [5]

Why Is High Quality Fish Oil So Important?

In March of 2010 in the state of California a lawsuit was filed against some of the top consumer market supplement companies claiming they were knowingly selling fish oil supplements contaminated with high levels of toxic polychlorinated biphenyl (PCB) compounds. This toxic contamination is despite claims on the label that the products have been treated and are safe from PCB contamination. [6][7]

Why Is This Important?

PCB contamination is linked to:
- Birth Defects
- Cancers of liver, skin, brain, and breast
- Hormonal problems

- Infertility
- Breast milk contamination

Bargain basement, and even many of the more expensive EPA-DHA fish oil concentrates on the consumer market scare me for these reasons:
- Rancidity
- Toxic contamination
- Low potency
- Some don't contain what they claim
- Some are made from the left-overs of cat food production.
- Many just don't get the job done.

I have learned the hard way that the most expensive supplement is the one that doesn't work

You risk damaging your health. In many cases, you are better off taking nothing rather than consuming a contaminated, rancid product.

You miss the opportunity and benefit from effective, quality supplementation.

You risk discouragement and "giving up" on a crucially important piece of your Wellness and Healing.

The Omega EPA-DHA concentrate products that I find work best in clinical practice are:
- *Omega 820 Pro* for highest potency and effectiveness
- *Omega Pure Liquid Pro* for those who struggle with swallowing capsules
- *Omega 780 EC Pro* is enterically coated to help those who have burping problems with fish oil supplementation

For most people, 2/meal of the *Omega 820 Pro* 2X/day is a start. For many, especially if their Essential Fatty Acid test levels are very low, 6/day makes sense. For some with autoimmune disease, 9/day can be quite helpful. It is important to note, that for smokers and those with high oxidative stress, EPA-DHA supplements can be oxidized and go rancid too easily in the body. For some, we must clean up their LifeStyle, help them detoxify, and restore anti-oxidant defenses before *Omega 820 Pro* supplementation can be safe and effective.

Core3: ***Vitamin D-3 5000 Pro*** – almost everyone tests suboptimum on this critical regulator of cell energy and health. D-3 5000 Pro supports:

- Reduced pain and inflammation
- Reduced cardiovascular risk
- Reduced high blood pressure
- Improved blood sugar and insulin regulation for those with Type 1 & 2 diabetes
- Prevention and management of arthritis and inflammatory diseases

- Reduction of multiple sclerosis incidence and symptoms
- Improvements in depression and SAD (Seasonal Affective Disorder)
- Improvement in epilepsy symptoms
- Reduced aches and pain
- Improvement in migraine headaches
- Improvement with infertility problems
- Reduced risk of many types of cancer
- Natural antibiotic effects through up-regulating your production of potent anti-microbial peptides
- Prevention and management of osteoporosis
- Improvement in prostate symptoms
- Decreases pain in neuropathy and fibromyalgia.
- Production of neurons in memory centers of our brain.

Extensive lab testing of Vitamin D blood levels (25-OH Vitamin D-3 blood test through LabCorp is best) has taught me that over 90% of everyone I test in Arizona is suboptimal in their Vitamin D blood levels. I shudder to think what was like in Minnesota where I practiced for 21 years before this testing was available. If you think you get enough Vitamin D from the sun or your diet, think again.

I now assume low Vitamin D until proven otherwise. At two of my recent post-graduate educational conferences, the medical physician presenters stated that the time is coming when it will be considered medical malpractice to fail to test, supplement, and monitor Vitamin D levels – it is that important!

Vitamin D and Bone Health

The mass media keep pounding us with the message that calcium is the key to bone health. Not true. Have we been enjoying declining rates of osteoporosis as we have elevated our calcium supplementation? Instead, we have one of the highest osteoporosis rates of any country in the world. So what are we missing?

Vitamin D3 controls our calcium absorption or uptake. Vitamin D3, when optimized to our ideal blood levels increases your calcium absorption and uptake 30 fold! Vitamin D, not calcium supplements, is crucial to optimizing our calcium levels for bone health. The tiny amounts of Vitamin D in most calcium supplements is not nearly enough to optimize Vitamin D blood levels. My past 9 years of Vitamin D3 blood testing have shown that virtually everyone needs much more.

Calcium supplements typically contain 800 IU of Vitamin D. In practice, I use 5000 IU size Vitamin D3 capsules and find that most people need 2 -6 of these 5000 IU capsules each day to optimize their blood Vitamin D-3 levels – that is 10,000 – 30,000 IU's daily.

There is a risk to optimizing our calcium levels for bone health – calcification of our arteries, joints, and soft tissues. Vitamin K plays a crucial role in keeping us safe from this dangerous calcification. This is discussed in detail later in this chapter under the Vitamin K section.

Can You Overdose Vitamin D?

Everything has a toxic dose – including water (drowning) and oxygen (hyperoxia). What we learned in the past about "dangerous Vitamin D" is mostly incorrect. It was related to medical prescription of Vitamin D-2 which is synthetic and dangerous and I NEVER recommend Vitamin D-2.

Vitamin D-3, the natural form is unlikely to cause toxicity at doses under 40,000 IU/day for the general population. In the largest study of its type on Vitamin D, researchers concluded that Vitamin D-3 Blood levels in the 60-80 ng/ml range were needed to reduce cancer risk and toxicity did not start until 200 ng/ml. (8)

There is a wide range of safety for Vitamin D-3 and our current understanding is reversed from what I was taught 28 years ago. Too little Vitamin D-3 is dangerous, and too much Vitamin D-3 is the lesser concern.

The real concern with overdoing Vitamin D-3 is an elevated blood calcium level above 10.2. Balance is the goal. Ideal blood levels of Vitamin D-3, in my experience, are 75-150 ng/ml. For some, this happens with as little as 4000 IU, for others, 45,000 IU/day may be needed for 8-12 weeks followed by a daily maintenance dose of as high as 30,000 IU/day.

This is due to many factors including: genetic Single Nucleotide Polymorphisms (SNP's) – genetic defects affecting Vitamin D utilization, mal-absorption, poor conversion to its active form in the liver, poor conversion to its active form in the kidney etc. Because of this, virtually everyone needs a routine 25-OH Vitamin D-3 blood test. In practice, I routinely do this budget-friendly, affordable test for almost everyone.

To raise levels when they are deficient or sub-optimum, the Vitamin D supplements I find work best are:
- *D3 5000 Pro* for high potency, easy to swallow capsules
- *Ultra D-3 5000 Pro* for easy to swallow capsules
- *D3 Liquid Pro* for those who struggle to swallow even small capsules

Core4: Magnesium Citrate Pro - essential for energy, metabolism, weight management, heart health, and staying well. *Magnesium Citrate Pro* supports:
- Cellular energy production
- Calm, peaceful, balance of your nervous system
- Reduced muscle spasm and restless legs
- Natural and safe lowering of high blood pressure
- Reduced heart arrhythmia problems
- Heart health and reduced angina symptoms
- Increased HDL (good cholesterol)
- Reduced blood clot, heart attack, and stroke risk
- Improved bowel function – especially helps most constipation
- Mood balance and depression relief

- Strong bones and improvements with osteoporosis
- Insomnia relief – magnesium is essential for great sleep!
- Prevention of kidney stones
- PMS relief (and sometimes cravings for chocolate)
- Raynaud's and limb circulation improvements
- Improvements with dry skin
- Reduction in seizures

Note: Do not take high-potency magnesium supplements with oils or fats or meals. Here is how to take magnesium to maximize absorption and benefits:

1. Start at (1) capsule of *Magnesium Citrate Pro* before bed and again (1) capsule in the AM 15 or more minutes before breakfast.
2. Increase to (2) capsules of *Magnesium Citrate Pro* before bed and again (2) capsules in the AM 15 or more minutes before breakfast.
3. Increase to (3) capsules of *Magnesium Citrate Pro* before bed and again (3) capsules in the AM 15 or more minutes before breakfast.
4. Increase to (4) capsules of *Magnesium Citrate Pro* before bed and again (4) capsules in the AM 15 or more minutes before breakfast.
5. Increase to (5) capsules of *Magnesium Citrate Pro* before bed and again (5) capsules in the AM 15 or more minutes before breakfast.
6. Increase to (6) capsules of *Magnesium Citrate Pro* before bed and again (6) capsules in the AM 15 or more minutes before breakfast.

Note: Reduce dose when you reach the threshold dose creating loose stools or diarrhea to normalize your bowels. If loose stools or diarrhea occurs before reaching 4 caps PM and 4 caps AM, you likely have some mal-absorption problems. We then recommend you switch to *MagnesiumGlycinate Pro* for enhanced absorption using same loading dose instructions above.

Is Magnesium Supplementation Safe?

Magnesium is one of the safest supplements available. Too much creates a laxative effect (think Milk of Magnesia laxative) so you simply flush through what you can't absorb. The time for concern with Magnesium safety is late stage kidney failure (near dialysis) or for those on kidney dialysis.

Magnesium deficiency IS DANGEROUS however. This is a concern since 80% of our population is deficient. (9)

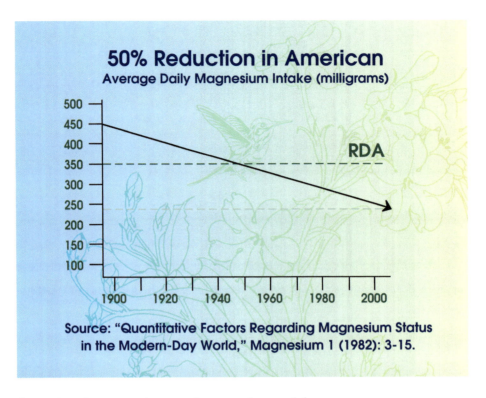

Source: "Quantitative Factors Regarding Magnesium Status in the Modern-Day World," Magnesium 1 (1982): 3-15.

In clinical practice, the magnesium supplements that work best are:
- *MagCitrate Pro* for those with normal bowel function or for those with constipation
- *MagnesiumGlycinate Pro* for those with malabsorption issues or a tendency towards diarrhea
- Topically applied magnesium oil for those who still need more magnesium
- Taurine to help your body hold onto magnesium. Many people, especially when under stress, waste magnesium by urinating it out of their bodies.

Probiotic Supplementation

If I were to add a 5th supplement to the Core 4, the top of my list would be a safe, effective Probiotic. What does *probiotic* mean? *Pro* means for. *Biotic* means life. *For life, health, and Wellness* is a fitting description for probiotics.

Probiotic supplements are friendly bacteria to support balance and health in our gut. Our microflora are the bacteria that live in our gut – friendly and unfriendly. For health, we need lots of happy, friendly bacteria to keep the disease and sickness causing unfriendly bacteria in check – like a healthy lawn chokes out weeds to keep them in control.

CHAPTER 5 PAGE 83

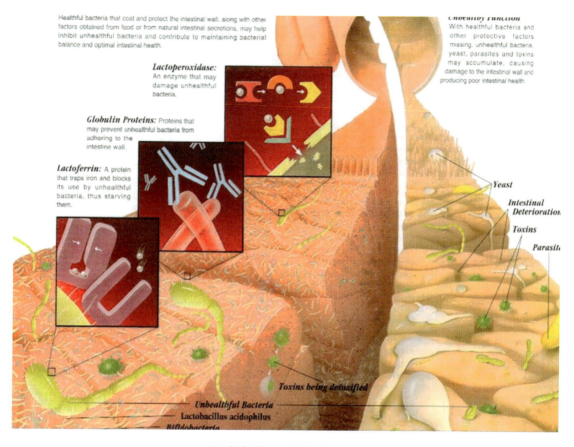

Graphic kindly provided by Metagenics

Notice lots of healthy bacteria on left side of diagram blocking the ability of the unhealthy, green-colored bacteria(microbes) to attach to wall of the gut creating damage.

On the right side of diagram, we see unhealthy bacteria damaging and destroying the crucial inner lining or our gut that protects us from microbes and their toxins.

Here is What You Need to Know About Your Microflora

- Your gut microflora, contains 20 trillion bacteria (that's 20X the number of cells in your body) and weighs 5 lbs. in a typical adult. It is one of our largest organs.
- Our microflora can make us fat, toxic, and sick when out of balance.
- You can have problems with your microflora – too many harmful bacteria and not enough friendly, health promoting bacteria with NO Digestive or Gut Symptoms! You may struggle with losing weight, fatigue, or any of a long list of symptoms and diseases.

Probiotics play a role in:
- Neurotransmitter production and regulation.
- Brain and mood balance. (see Brain-Gut connection graphic on page 33)
- Our Western Lifestyles make it hard to keep your microflora and digestive systems healthy.
- The healing process for Leaky Gut and our microflora can take longer than previously understood - and some never get well without effective help.
- Getting your gut and microflora assessed is a smart investment in your health and Wellness.

So Why Different Probiotics?

We have over 500 different bacteria types identified so far in our gut. It is essential to use only the potent, effective probiotic strains that have been clinically tested in humans and work in real life. Few of the probiotics on the consumer market have this testing and far too many work in the test tube, but not in your gut. Some even change in the human gut to pathogenic or carcinogenic strains. Probiotics of dubious researched quality and safety scare me.

ONLY USE PROBIOTICS WITH A PEDIGREE

A safe probiotic is listed in collection of American cultures: it has the name of the strain of probiotic followed by a list of numbers – like a pedigree. No pedigree and is like buying a dog off the street – you have no idea of what you are really getting. This is what a safe probiotic strain history looks like:

Probiotic Max Restore Pro Strain History

Probiotic Strains: (Note: Each strain in this professional-grade product was selected because of proven safety, tolerance, resistance to bile and acidity, survival in the GI tract, and no contribution to antibiotic resistance.)

HOWARU® Biff (Bifidobacterium lactis HN019): Researchers have identified Bifidobacterium lactis HN019 as having the best probiotic potential among more than 2,000 strains. Its adherence in high numbers to cultured intestinal epithelial cells, contributes to its ability to modulate immunity. Preservation or restoration of healthy intestinal microbiotia by this strain have been demonstrated. In middle-aged to elderly people Bifidobacterium lactis HN019 increased cytotoxic activity of NK cells and phagocytic activity of peripheral blood mononucleocytes and was non- inflammatory. In a year-long, double-blind, placebo-controlled trial (n-600), children (aged 1-3) receiving this strain along with galacto-oligosaccharides showed improved immunity, iron status, and growth. In a 14 day study (n= 100), B. lactis HN019 proved to dose-dependently increase colon transit time and reduce frequency of digestive complaints.

Lactobacillus acidophilus (Lactobacillus acidophilus La-14): This common inhabitant of the human mouth, intestinal tract, and vagina has diverse health benefits. In vitro studies indicate that L. acidophilus La-14 has excellent adhesion to human epithelial celllines (HT-29), limiting the ability of enteric pathogens to colonize. This vancomycin-sensitive strain has shown inhibition of common bacterialstrains in vitro, and re-establishment of the population of lactobacillus and bifidobacterium in the intestinal tracts of mice after antibiotic therapy. L. acidophilus La-14 has been demonstrated to support specific immunity in humans, shifting the immune system to the Th1 response (induced IL-12 and moderately induced TNF-a in vitro). It degrades oxalate 100%.

Lactobacillus plantarum (Lactobacillus plantarum Lp-115): Isolated from plant material, this strain is abundantly present in lactic acid-fermented foods such as olives and sauerkraut. In vitro studies have shown that L.plantarum Lp-115 has excellent adhesion to epithelial cell lines. In vitro, this strain degraded oxalates 40% and either inhibited adhesion or displaced a variety of common pathogens. These studies support the notion that the strain shifts the immune response to the Th 1 type. In animal models, L. plantarum Lp-115 reduced gut inflammation. Bifidobacterium longum (Bifidobacterium longum B1-05): B.longum B1-05 is well suited to the intestinal environment. It is sensitive to vancomycin.

Saccharomyces boulardii (Sb) is a natural, non-pathogenic yeast that has been shown to maintain and restore the healthy ecology of the small and large intestines. In a 2010 systematic review and meta-analysis of 31 randomized, placebo-controlled treatment arms in 27 trials (encompassing 5029 adult study patients), S. Boulardii was found to be significantly efficacious and safe in 84% of those treatments arms. Extensively researched and published in European and American peer-reviewed journals, Saccharomyces boulardii has demonstrated multiple mechanisms of action. (Note: Saccharomyces boulardii is the yeast that kills pathogenic yeast like Candida overgrowth)

The Saccharomyces boulardii used in this formula is processed by drying at a controlled temperature and low vacuum for improved stability.

References for *Probiotic Max Restore Pro* *(10-29)*

You won't find this history of effectiveness and safety in your bargain basement brands, most vitamin shops, and even most quality brands. Using anything less than this frightens me – to use personally or to recommend to my patients.

The reason I have invested in extensive training and the clinical evaluation of the supplements we use is that the most expensive – and sometimes dangerous – supplements are those that don't work. You lose money, time, and the opportunity to get well and often become discouraged and give up – a sad waste all around.

So What Works?

Supplementing with Probiotics is not a cure-all. To work effectively, we need to clean up our LifeStyle and if needed, go through the "4R" program described in Chapter 1.

For many, *prebiotics* are also important for success. Prebiotics are like "fertilizer" to support the Probiotic "grass seeds" in creating a healthy "lawn" or microecology in the gut.

For others, Immunoglobulin support is needed to promote health and balance of our gut immune system. Antibiotics, sickness, junk food and many other things can disrupt this delicate balance. Remember, almost 80% of our immune system is around our gut so it profoundly affects our whole body health, balance, and Wellness.

The combination product that I find works best initially in clinical practice for most is *Probiotic Max Restore Pro* with it's strain history described in the previous pages. It is a wonderful combination for repair of leaky gut and restoration of gut health.

Probiotic Max Restore Pro contains multiple clinically effective probiotic strains, prebiotics (the arabinogalactans), and therapeutic levels of viable Saccharomyces (The friendly yeast that kills unfriendly yeast). It contains a wonderful blend of Immunoglobulins to support "cleaning house" in your gut and a return to immune balance.

The straight probiotic formula that I like best is the highly potent *Intestinal Probiotic 100 Billion Pro*. 100 Billion active colony forming units per capsule may sound like a lot but remember there are 20 trillion bacteria in our gut. These strains are similar to those in *Probiotic Max Restore Pro* which are extensively tested in clinical trials for safety and effectiveness.

Intestinal Probiotic 100 Billion Pro does lack the potent anti-yeast *Saccharomyces boulardii* and the prebiotics that are present in *Probiotic Max Restore Pro.*

A great Prebiotic and therapeutic fiber combination that I really like to calm down an inflamed gut is *Intestinal Balance Pro*. Also *Gut Restore Pro* is often really helpful creating initial relief quickly.

A blend of InflamClear Pro, Gut Restore Pro, and Intestinal Balance Pro has been effective many times for me in practice for those with severe gut inflammation and even bleeding colitis. The recent availability of Probiotic Max Restore Pro to add to this blend makes it even better.

What About Iodine?

Iodine is critically linked to thyroid function. We have increasing thyroid disease problems like:
- Hypothyroidism
- Thyroid Nodules
- Autoimmune thyroiditis
- Hashimoto's thyroid disease
- 13 million thyroid disease sufferers and growing

Thyroid Insufficiency Symptoms

- Fatigue
- Low metabolism
- Weight gain/fat gain
- Dry skin or hair
- Sensitivity to cold
- Constipation
- Low basal body temperature

Why So Many Thyroid Problems?

For your thyroid to make T4 or thyroid hormone, you need plenty of iodine. To convert T4 to the much more active T3, you need plenty of zinc and selenium. For your cell receptors to be sensitive so that they can respond properly to active thyroid hormone (T3), you also need plenty of Vitamins A and D.

Our thyroid gland is a sentinel gland to toxic chemicals and heavy metals. For many, thyroid problems signal excess toxic load.

So you see the problem - lots of things to go wrong affecting your thyroid gland. Let's take just Iodine.

"…19-23% of women between ages of 30 and 60 years were iodine deficient. Thus, iodine deficiency is again becoming significant, especially in women in the United States." [30]

In addition to our iodine deficiency problems, many suffer from suboptimal zinc, selenium, Vitamin D, or Vitamin A. Excessive stress impairs the conversion of T4 to active T3 and increase reverse T3 which blocks T3 activity. In short, vitamin and mineral deficiencies, toxic load, and excessive stress mess up your thyroid function.

In my clinical experience, the vast majority of "thyroid" problems are secondary. This means the thyroid is not the problem – the thyroid gland is just responding normally to toxic load, nutritional deficiencies, and excessive stress. Fixing the causes, not treating the thyroid is the approach that works best and avoids lots of side effects.

Are You Getting Enough Iodine?

Iodine is needed for:
- Balanced thyroid activity
- Proper growth and development
- Normal metabolism
- Healthy reproductive function
- Estrogen receptor sensitivity to help avoid:
  - Fibrocystic breast disease
  - Elevated breast, prostate, and ovarian cancer risk

Iodine Recommendations

- RDI – 120-150 mcg for adults = .003% optimum
- Optimum – 25-50 mg Iodine/Iodide at ratio of .66/1

Notice the huge difference between Optimum and RDI (recommended daily intake). The RDI is newer and replaces the old RDA (recommended daily allowance). Remember 1 mg = 1000 mcg. This means the RDI for Iodine is far too low. Use caution with increasing Iodine intake too quickly if autoimmune thyroid disease is an issue.

At a recent conference, the presenter referred to the RDI as a "really dumb idea". In the case of iodine, the presenter was right. Remember that the RDI is the minimum amount needed to prevent deficiency disease for a general population. It says almost nothing about our individual needs with our unique genetics, lifestyle, mal-absorption issues, stress and toxic load.

Healthy populations with much less thyroid disease than ours such as Japan and Okinawa consume between 12mg and 200 mg of Iodine from seafood and kelp daily. In America, the average is 240 micrograms. This means that the Japanese, who have one of the lowest breast cancer rates in the world, consume almost 50X more Iodine than Americans who have the highest incidence of breast cancer in the world. Of course there is more than just Iodine involved in our 1st place rating for breast cancer, but low Iodine levels are appear to be quite important. (31-36)

What About Vitamin K?

Vitamin K is a fat-soluble vitamin that is most well-known for the important role it plays in blood clotting. The "K" is for the German word "Klot" since it was discovered by a German. However, Vitamin K also essentials roles in:

- Building strong bones and preventing osteoporosis
- Preventing hardening of our arteries and heart disease
- Preventing Alzheimer's dementia and may help to manage this disease
- Vitamin K in topical form may help to reduce bruising
- Vitamin K appears to help Metabolic Syndrome by supporting insulin and blood sugar regulation which may be helpful for those with diabetes and pre-diabetes
- Vitamin K appears to have antioxidant properties and works with Vitamin D to help control a multitude of our genetic pathways essential for health and Wellness

It is so important that you should seriously consider adding Vitamin K in supplemental form because most people do not get nearly enough Vitamin K on a daily basis through the leafy green veggies or other foods they eat.

In fact, Vitamin K is sometimes referred to as "the forgotten vitamin" because its major benefits are often overlooked. Following are some important facts about vitamin K that will highlight its critical role in your health and Wellness. (37)

Which is Best Type of Vitamin K?

Vitamin K1 is found naturally in plants and aids in normal clotting. Getting extra Vitamin K does not necessarily make you clot excessively. There are exceptions - if you are taking the blood clot inhibiting medication Coumadin or Warfarin, Vitamin K1 and to a lesser degree Vitamin K-2 supplementation can reduce the effectiveness of these drugs. Also, if you have a history of serious blood clots, heart attacks, or strokes, consult your physician before starting Vitamin K supplementation.

Vitamin K2 is made by the bacteria that live in our gastrointestinal tract if we have a healthy gut bacterial balance. The MK-7 version of this is what is what I usually recommend. At low levels, it does appear safe for those who take Coumadin or Warfarin. This will be discussed further below.

Vitamin K3 is a synthetic form that lacks many of the benefits of K1 and K2. Toxicity can happen with this injectable, synthetic version and I never recommend it.

Which Type of Vitamin K2 Is Best?

MK4 is a synthetic form very similar to Vitamin K1. Unfortunately, MK4 has a very short half-life of about one hour making it a poor dietary supplement. After being absorbed from your gut, the MK4 version of Vitamin K2 remains mostly in your liver aiding in the production of blood-clotting factors. This type of Vitamin K is the greatest concern for those taking blood thinner medications like Coumadin or Warfarin.

MK7 is a newer form of Vitamin K2 that is much more effective because it stays in your body longer remaining active for almost three days. It also has a smaller effect on blood clotting and a larger role in reducing dangerous calcification of our arteries.

In our clinic and store, I recommend *Vitamin K2 Pro*, which is a natural form and not toxic at even 500 times the RDI. Vitamin K2 as the preferred MK7 form is also available in the fermented food natto. The supplement, *Nattokinase*, used to improve blood flow has its Vitamin K removed.

Vitamin K2 as the MK7 form in *Vitamin K2 Pro* is the preferred Vitamin K for most of the patients I see. I reserve the use of Vitamin K1 for those who have poor clotting and easy bruising problems.

Vitamin K Prevents Hardening of Your Arteries

Vitamin K has an important role in keeping calcium in our bones – and out of our soft tissues. When we lack sufficient Vitamin K, calcium can leave our bones and be deposited in our artery lining leading to hardening of our arteries. We can also experience calcification of our artery plaque creating further problems.

In addition, Vitamin K appears to have a role in keeping calcium from leaving our bones and depositing in our joints as bone spurs and in our kidneys as kidney stones.

Of special importance is the apparent risk of increased calcification of arteries and joints when using high-dose Vitamin D supplementation without sufficient extra Vitamin K.

Vitamin D and Vitamin K work together to increase MGP which works to protect your blood vessels from calcification. MGP is so important that it is used as a laboratory measure of your blood vessel and heart health. Low levels of MGP appear linked to increased calcification or hardening of our arteries – including the coronary arteries supplying blood to our heart. (38)

High dose Vitamin D3 supplementation is good for your bones through increasing our blood calcium levels. This is not, however, so beneficial for your arteries which can become calcified. *Vitamin K2, as MK 7 form, shines for its ability to protect our arteries from calcification or hardening as we raise blood calcium levels with extra Vitamin D3. Remember, Vitamin D3, when optimized to ideal blood levels increases your calcium absorption and uptake 30 fold!*

For this reason, I include Vitamin K2 Pro supplementation with high dose (over 15,000IU/day) Vitamin D for most of my patients.

Build Strong Bones to Prevent Osteoporosis

Vitamin K is one of the most important nutritional supplements for improving bone density. When used with optimal levels of Vitamin D (using blood testing) and Bone Build Pro (bone matrix) and Regenerix Pro (a bioavailable silica source), we have seen patients reverse osteoporosis to normal in as little as 12 months.

Absorbing Vitamin K

Vitamin K deficiency can also be related to mal-absorption. Dietary fat is needed to absorb this fat soluble vitamin. This means that in order for your body to absorb Vitamin K effectively, you need to eat some fat along with it, have effective fat digestion, and effective fat absorption. If you struggle with "leaky gut", low stomach acid, gall bladder problems, or insufficient pancreatic digestive enzymes, you are likely insufficient in multiple fat soluble vitamins including Vitamin K, Vitamin D, Vitamin A, and Vitamin E.

One easy way to supply healthy fats to aid Vitamin K, Vitamin D, Vitamin A, and Vitamin E absorption is by taking with our *Omega 820 Pro* fish oil concentrate with our fat soluble vitamins. Adding Digest Boost Pro for stomach acid support and Digest Enzyme Boost Pro for extra fat digestive support can also be helpful. This will help ensure that our Vitamin K is well-absorbed by our body.

Safety of Vitamin K

Some have the erroneous belief that Vitamin K is dangerous because it promotes clotting and too much clotting creates blocked blood flow to our legs, lung, heart, or brain. Remember our definition of health - **health = balance**.

Too *much* clotting is indeed dangerous. Too *little* clotting is also dangerous because we can bleed out or hemorrhage – sometimes fatally. We desire balance for health and Wellness.

This being said, there is **no known toxicity** associated with high doses of the Vitamin K1 (phylloquinone) or Vitamin K2 (menaquinone) (39)

Vitamin K Does Not Cause Blood Clots

The same is not true for injectable, synthetic menadione (vitamin K_3). Synthetic Vitamin K-3 (menadione) given by injection has caused toxicity and is no longer used for treatment of vitamin K deficiency.

So What Causes Too Much Clotting?

There are strong links between inflammation and hypercoagulability (too much clotting). What causes this increased inflammation activating the excessive clotting or coagulability?
- Excessive toxicity or toxin overload
- Allergy – especially delayed food allergies
- Excessive stress and release of cortisol and other stress hormones
- Chronic low-grade infections – not usually detected with usual medical tests
- Nutrient depletion – especially of essential fatty acids, Vitamins D, and Vitamin E
- Genetic predisposition combined with a LifeStyle that doesn't fit your genetic needs. (40)

How Do We Measure This?

Fibrinogen is one inexpensive blood lab marker. Fibrinogen is synthesized in the liver and circulates in the blood. At the time of injury or inflammation, fibrinogen is converted to fibrin, which is the material that forms blood clots. A fibrinogen blood test measures the levels of fibrinogen in your blood. High blood fibrinogen levels indicate increased inflammation or injury, increased clotting risk, and increased risk to coronary heart disease.

The ISAC panel through Hemex labs is also quite helpful to understand the genetic "weakspots" behind hypercoagulabilty. (41)

Nutrient and Drug Interactions with Vitamin K (42)

Vitamin A and Vitamin E have been found to increase need for Vitamin K. (43) Large doses of Vitamin A appears to reduce Vitamin K absorption. A form of Vitamin E metabolite may inhibit vitamin K-dependent enzyme activity. One study in adults found that supplementation with 1,000 IU of Vitamin E for 12 weeks decreased Vitamin K-dependent protein activity. (43) Vitamin E at 1,200IU daily has been reported to inhibit Vitamin K activity which combined with taking anticoagulatory drugs resulted in excessive bleeding. (44)

Some Food Sources of Vitamin K

- Collard Greens
- Spinach
- Salad Greens
- Kale
- Broccoli
- Brussel Sprouts
- Cabbage

Who Needs Extra Vitamin K?

Those with a personal or family history of:
- Osteoporosis
- Hardening of the arteries - arteriosclerosis
- Artery disease – atherosclerosis, aneurysms
- Heart disease
- Too much fast food and not enough leafy, green vegetables
- Digestive disease – Crohn's, ulcerative Colitis, celiac, leaky gut, mal-digestion, mal-absorption
- Liver disease
- Drug use especially antibiotics, cholesterol lowering drugs, and aspirin

How Much Vitamin K is Right For Me?

Although each person is different one vitamin K expert, Dr. Cees Vermeer, recommends between 45 mcg and 185 mcg of vitamin K2 daily for most adults. I suggest 45 mcg of *Vitamin K2 Pro* daily twice daily as a starting point for most. If mal-digestion, mal-absorption, and leaky gut are an issue, I may recommend 45 mcg. of *Vitamin K2 Pro* three times daily with digestive enzyme and stomach acid supplement support.

You must use caution on the higher doses if you take anticoagulants. For those on Coumadin or Warfarin, *Vitamin K2 Pro* appears to have an effect on blood thinning medications at levels of 50mcg or more/day. Since one *Vitamin K-2 Pro* contains 45mcg, one per day appears to be safe for those on blood thinners. Also, when taken consistently, Vitamin K-2 (MK-7) may result in a more stable INR (45)

Who Should Not Take Vitamin K Without Consulting Their Physician?

Pregnant and nursing mothers should avoid vitamin K supplemental intakes higher than the RDI (65 mcg) unless specifically recommended and monitored by their physician. Those who have experienced stroke, heart attack, or serious blood clots should not take vitamin K without first consulting their physician.

To learn more about Vitamin K, see the references in reference section at back of this book. (46-57)

Which Supplements Can Help Me Handle Stress?

My first choice is usually magnesium. For some patients I will substitute *CNS Relax Max Pro* for *Magnesium Citrate Pro* in the Core 4 – with others I add this to the Core 4. I have had surprising success helping patients become more peaceful and overall balanced with *CNS Relax Max Pro*.

CNS Relax Max Pro integrates the synergistic benefits of magnesium, myoinositol, L-taurine, GABA, and L-theanine. Because it works upstream to delicately rebalance 1st and 2nd messenger signaling pathways, it creates a wide range of benefits.

Some of the benefits we see clinically with *CNS Relax Max Pro*:
- Drops cravings and cortisol (your main stress hormone)
- Neuronal and hormonal stabilization – helps balance nerves and hormones
- Increased estrogen, ovarian function, and HDL
- Decreased triglycerides, body mass, and leptin
- Decreased glutamate exitotoxicity
- L-theanine in this product helps hold on to taurine which helps to hold on to magnesium
- Reduces lipid peroxidation and oxidative stress
- Lowers homocysteine
- Anti-inflammatory protection - an antidote for excessive inflammation activation
- Improves mitochondrial energy production and decreases free radical production
  - Important for arrhythmias and cardiomyopathy
  - Highly important in nephropathy, retinopathy, cataract formation, neuropathy
  - Improves glucose utilization and decreases HgA1C lab marker
  - Supports improved insulin sensitivity
  - Helpful with catabolism(muscle loss) and fatigue

So how do we explain such a wide range of benefits?

Think of a fire in your kitchen that has grown to flames 6 feet high. What does it take to put it out? LOTS of water, fire extinguisher foam, and effort are required - lots of side effects. This is like using a powerful drug to put out inflammation in your nervous system when is blazing with heat – with lots of collateral damage and side-effects.

If you move way upstream to when the fire is just about to start, how much does it take to stop it - just a puff of air or a few ounces of water. Working to balance 1st and 2nd messenger signaling pathways is like whispering to balance a very complex system way upstream.

Which Supplements Do You Recommend for Bone Building?

What doesn't work is calcium – in fact the countries with the highest cow's milk and calcium intakes have the highest osteoporosis rates. The high acid dairy, soda, and junk food (and low veggie diets) of typical Americans creates an acid pH in the body which is buffered with calcium and other minerals from our bones – and then lost in our urine.

Countries like Japan with very low milk consumption have a small fraction of our osteoporosis problems. They get their essential minerals – including calcium – from whole grains, veggies, nuts and other whole foods.

Bone is not made of calcium – it is made of MANY minerals, micronutrients, and importantly, protein. Think of a 15 story office building. The steel beams of the building are like the collagen fibers of your bone. These "beams" make our bone both strong and flexible.

A key reason that the biphosphonate osteoporosis drugs work so poorly and have so many side effects is that they don't address the loss of the collagen protein "steel beams" that form the framework of healthy bone. These drugs slow the removal of old bone to make bone denser. Denser bone is not necessarily stronger. Like a piece of chalk your teacher used on the blackboard – very dense – what happens when it is dropped on the floor?

Healthy bone involves sufficient protein, ALL of the needed Vitamins, Minerals, and trace elements and balanced cellular messaging. If your body is on fire with inflammation, you melt away bone. If you are super-stressed or toxic, you melt away bone.

Our bone reflects our over-all health. When you are losing bone, you are losing muscle and other organ mass as well. Losing bone means you are catabolic – breaking down faster than you repair. This means your body is in accelerated aging – and eating you – like a cannibal.

The only effective way to restore bone health is to treat the whole person. That being said, along with normalizing gut function, sleep, exercise, detoxification, stress management, and eating smart to fit your needs, the following are some of my favorite products to prevent and reverse bone loss:

Nutrient Therapy – Bone Health

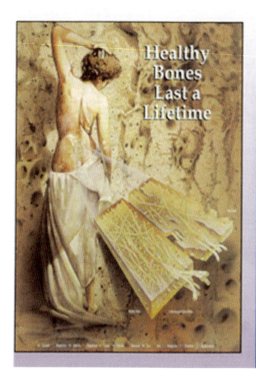

Bone Build Pro (58)
- Lead-free bone matrix
- Rich in multiple mineral co-factors
- Supports bone mineralization.
- Supports bone strength & flexibility
- Supports bone regeneration

Remember, bone is made of much more than just calcium!

Graphic kindly provided by Metagenics

<u>I almost NEVER recommend straight calcium supplements</u>. They don't work compared to bone matrix supplements that contain the complex mix of minerals needed for bone health. In fact, years of intracellular mineral testing has shown me that most people are far more deficient in magnesium, than calcium. This means that for many, they need magnesium more than calcium for healthy bones.

Most importantly, optimizing your Vitamin D levels increases calcium absorption from your food 30 fold! This means that a reasonable diet of fresh foods, whole grains, nuts and seeds is likely to supply plenty of calcium as long as your Vitamin D levels are optimized. For this reason – and many others, I recommend supplemental Vitamin D for almost everyone using blood Vitamin D-3 levels to optimize dosage.

For many with significant to severe bone loss problems, I also recommend:
- Vitamin K2 Pro to support bone health and minimize calcium transferring from our bones to our arteries causing hardening of the arteries. This calcium transfer from bone can also cause kidney stones, soft tissue calcification, and bone spurs. With higher dose Vitamin D-3 supplementation, it is important to add Vitamin K2 to prevent these problems. It also supports bone health by promoting carboxylation of bone proteins. (59-65)

- Regenerix Pro supports (66-71)
  - Reduces Fine Lines and Wrinkles
  - Thickens and Strengthens Hair
  - Strengthens Nails
  - Increases Hip Bone Mineral Density
  - Adds Flexibility to Bone
  - Promotes Healthy Joints

Last, but far from least, we must supply plenty of quality, bio-available amino acids (from protein) to build bone collagen "steel beams" for bone strength. **Complete Boost Pro** is my favorite Functional Food powder (makes a great tasting shake) for these reasons:
- Supports muscle and bone building
- Supports improved metabolism and fat loss
- Supports reduce inflammation
- Supports enhanced detoxification
- Supports intestinal health and healing
- Supports enhanced immune function

How Do I Know My Supplement Program Is Working For Me?

When your ICW (IntraCellular Water from chapter 1) is going up, your BCM (Body Cell Mass) is going up, and your Body Fat is going down, your supplement and LifeStyle program are working really well for you. When your LifeStyle score goes up, lab testing improves, and you report significant improvements in your health goals – like more energy and your clothes fit better, your care process is working really well for you.

By carefully monitoring objective findings (test and exam findings) as well as subjective findings (what you feel and self-rate), we can measure how your overall care program is working. It isn't just one supplement or one LifeStyle change to make a difference, it takes synergy between many factors for things to work for you. This is the reason for the book title, "*7 Secrets to Wellness*" – not just **one** Secret.

Why Does Physician-Grade Supplementation Matter?

It all boils down to: *Do you want what works?* Having tried to just send patients to buy supplements at stores or on the web, I learned quickly that not all supplements actually work in clinical practice. Here are some of the reasons:

ConsumerLab.com report finds unexpected nutrient levels, contamination.
By Jacqueline Stenson, MSNBC contributor,
msnbc.com updated 9:26 a.m. MT, Fri., Jan. 19, 2007

- "*Of 21 brands of multivitamins* on the market in the United States and Canada selected by ConsumerLab.com and tested by independent laboratories, just 10 met the stated claims on their labels or satisfied other quality standards."
- "Some did not dissolve in the correct amount of time, meaning they could potentially pass through the body without being fully absorbed."
- ConsumerLab.com announced today that its testing has shown that approximately "5% to 10% of certain mineral supplements are contaminated with lead."
- "*Half the products were fine, half were not,*" said Cooperman."
- *Most worrisome,*" according to ConsumerLab.com president Dr. Tod Cooperman, "is that one product, a *'Multivitamins Especially for Women'*, was contaminated with lead."

So how do you know if your supplement was "made in China" and is contaminated with lead, melamine, PCB's, pesticides, herbicides or rancid?

How do you know your supplement was not bottled in the back of someone's unsanitary garage with questionable ingredients?

How do you know if your supplement is formulated to be absorbable, bioavailable, synergistic, and effective in humans?

How do you know if your supplement really has what is claimed on the label?

You Don't!

Problems Discovered with Eight Vitamin D Supplements in Study by ConsumerLab.com

Incorrect Amounts of Vitamins, Lead Contamination, and Labeling Infractions Identified

White Plains, New York — April 26, 2010 — "Among 28 vitamin D supplements recently selected for independent testing, problems were found with 8 products, 29% of those reviewed", according to ConsumerLab.com

ConsumerLab.com Finds Quality Problems with Nearly Thirty Percent of Fish Oil Supplements Reviewed; "Fishy" Claims Identified

White Plains, New York – September 28, 2010 – "Tests of fish, algal and krill oil supplements revealed quality problems with 7 out of 24 products selected" by independent testing organization ConsumerLab.com.

ConsumerLab.com Finds Carcinogenic Form of Chromium in Supplements, Including Those for Weight Loss

White Plains, New York – March 2, 2010 — "A carcinogenic form of chromium, hexavalent chromium, is present is some dietary supplements", according to new tests by ConsumerLab.com.

For consumers and even skilled, experienced professionals, it can be a nightmare sorting through all the conflicting claims, slick marketing, and overload of choices.

At Renovare, we chose to invest in physician-grade supplements from reputable suppliers with 3rd party assays and on-site labs for quality assessment. Our suppliers and accountable to the physicians who use their products and evaluate patient response. Quality slips and the supplier is fired.

More than one company has disappeared from the physician-grade supplement market for just this reason. I have personally inspected the production facilities and the quality control processes of our major suppliers. They have:
- High tech labs to measure for contaminants, active ingredients, and potency.
  - When microbial contamination exceeds allowable limits, the batch of raw materials goes to the dump.
  - Most companies would overlook this or fail to test is the first place.
  - Many companies simply irradiate the raw materials to kill the microbial contaminants creating damage to active ingredients and other problems.
- They test the identity of the herbal compounds they receive to verify they are what they say they are. It is not uncommon to get the wrong herb from a supplier.
- The labs have machines to measure how quickly the tablets dissolve in a simulated stomach.
- They have special storage rooms to hold bottles from each batch to measure loss of potency over time. If they drop below label claim before expiration date, they are recalled and reformulated.

Are they more expensive? Yes, but not by as much as you might expect. Some "mass market" supplements even cost more than the physician-grade supplements. Time and time again patients come to me with bags of expensive mass market supplements. I ask, "Did they work for you?" Obviously not, or they wouldn't be in my office. The questions we must answer to help are:

- Which supplements do you need at this time?
- What dosage do you need now?
- How do we measure your response so we know what is working and what is not working for you?

We recommend only professional grade supplements because years of experience working with them have helped us determine which are likely to be effective in different situations. Then our job is to determine which fit your needs best and what dosage is most effective during the active treatment phase of your care.

When you complete your active care and graduate to maintenance care, your supplement program needs to again be fully revised. It is as important to know when to stop therapeutic dosage of different supplements as it is to know when to start. Too much or too little is harmful. More is not always better – everything has a toxic dose – even air and water. Remember, health is about balance.

Summary:

- Almost none of us get even the bare minimum or recommended daily intake (RDI) of all of our essential vitamins, minerals, and nutrients.
- Our stressful lifestyles, fast food, gut problems, and toxic load further increases our needs.
- Our pandemic of chronic disease is caused in part by deficiencies or being sub-optimum in these key vitamins, minerals, and nutrients.
- Supplementing Smart is a crucial part of creating a LifeStyle supporting our Wellness.
- An ounce of prevention through supplementing smart is worth more than many pounds of cure.
- Everyone is different so our supplement program needs to fit our unique needs – and change as we change.
- Testing is available to assess our needs and monitor our response to our supplement program.
- Supplements are a "supplement" to eating smart and do NOT replace smart eating.
- Effective, pure, safe supplements that actually work as intended and fit our needs are not so easy to find.
- **The most expensive supplements are the ones that don't work!**

Secret 6

Exercising Smart

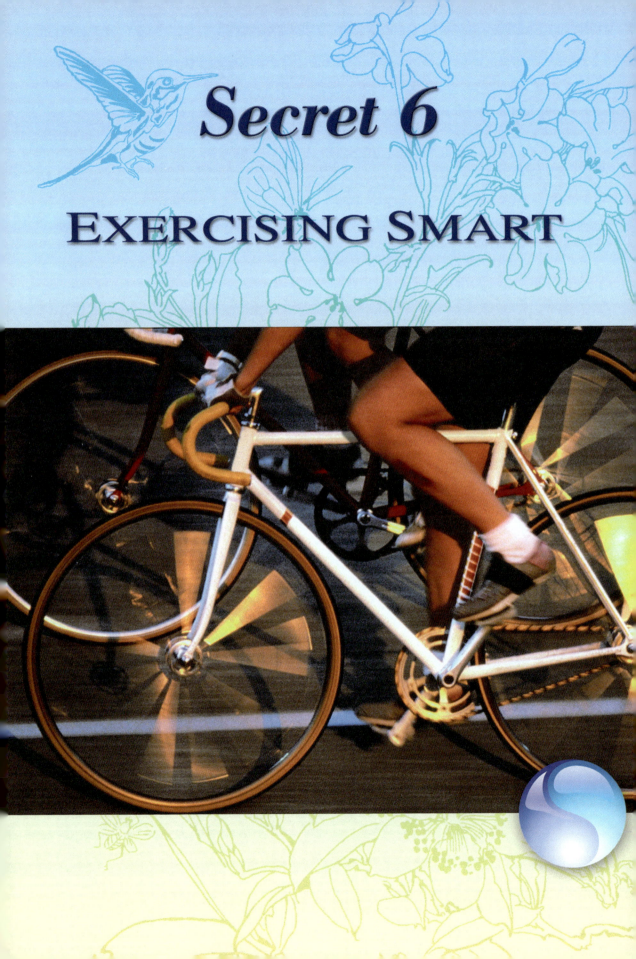

Chapter 6 Snapshot

- The key to energy, losing weight effectively (losing only fat), metabolism repair, and successful aging is gaining muscle mass (amount) and muscle strength.
- We need a combination of aerobic exercise, flexibility, and resistance exercise (strength training) to be fit and well.
- Almost all of the patients I see are lacking in effective resistance exercise to help build muscle mass and strength.
- For most, exercise alone is not enough to repair metabolism, support fat loss, and gain muscle and strength - the other 7 Secrets to Wellness must be addressed for exercise to be effective.
- We need to make exercise fun and a scheduled part of our LifeStyle to really work for the long-haul.
- Having a skilled trainer or coach is essential for most to get this done.

What Are The Best Biomarkers of Healthy (or Successful) Aging?

1. Your muscle mass (amount of muscle)
2. Your muscle strength [1]
3. Your blood sugar and insulin regulation (Chapter 1)

Exercise helps all 3!
Why?

Your long-term Health and Wellness are determined, more than almost anything else by the following:

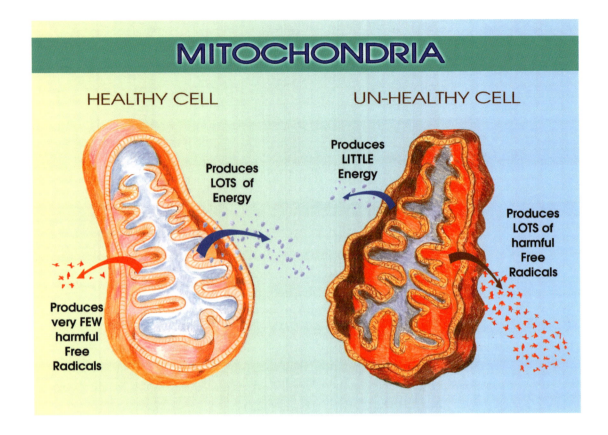

Can you guess what this is?

It's the engine that powers you! In your body, it's called a mitochondria and it is the engine or powerhouse for your cells. It converts food to energy and when it works well, you have lots of energy, few damaging free radicals and inflammation, and great metabolism so you burn calories instead of storing them as fat.

Guess which tissues are richest in mitochondria?

Muscle, especially in your heart muscle, as well as nerve cells (neurons) in your brain contain up to 2000 of these mitochondrial power houses within each microscopic cell.

Think "3M's":

1. **Mitochondia**
2. **Metabolism**
3. **Muscle**

They are all related. If you want to improve your health and Wellness, slow down aging, feel great, burn fat, you must increase the "3M's".

We use the amount of your body cell mass (muscle and organ mass rich in mitochondria) and IntraCellular Water (ICW) - an indirect measure of your metabolism - to calculate your biologic age. Some people are 40 years of chronological age (chronological age=number of birthdays), but their body works like an 80 year old body (biologic age=age at which their body functions).

Others are 80 years of chronological age, but their body works like a 40 year old body (biologic age). Your LifeStyle, including your exercise, is the most important factor in your biologic age. Feel discouraged and ready to throw in the towel?

We have had patients reduce their biologic age by 4 years in as little as 4 weeks. From personal experience, I have regained my health after major chronic illness and currently enjoy a biologic age almost half of my chronologic age.

To get started, exercise is extremely important. Yes, there are special supplements to help boost mitochondrial biogenesis (making more new mitochondria) and boosting your metabolism. But, nothing works better than exercise and an active LifeStyle combined with the other 7 *Secrets to Wellness*.

Why Do We Have So Little Muscle?

When we "*diet*" and reduce calories, we typically burn muscle (the red stuff on the following picture) and gain body fat percentage (the yellow stuff on the following picture). This damages our metabolism. Then we do it again and again – until we have lost so much muscle that dieting doesn't work anymore! The "DIE" in *DIET* is the sound of our metabolism *dying*!

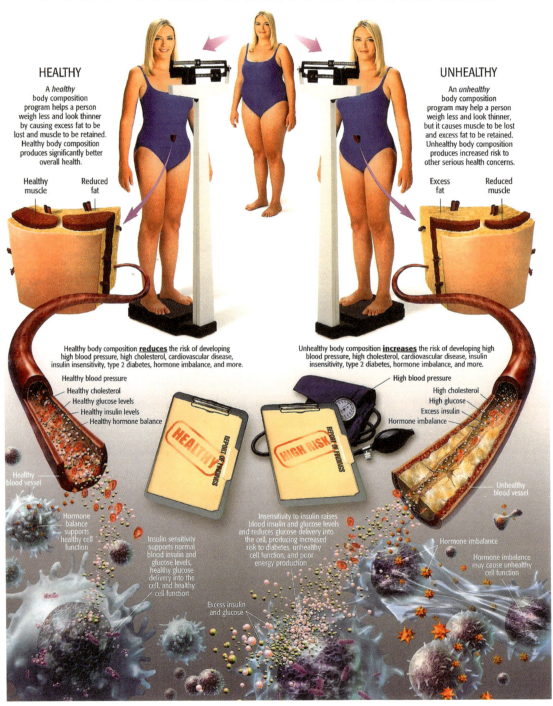

Graphic kindly provided by Metagenics

Typical dieting has unhealthy results as shown in the woman on the right. Do you really want to lose muscle, gain fat, and damage your metabolism and health so that you gain back the weight you lost – plus more -after you stop your diet? On top of this, what happens as we get older? We typically become less active. Exercise is pulling the chair up to the table, hoisting a drink, or operating the remote for our TV. We drive instead of walk and even use a golf cart to avoid walking the golf course. We lose muscle, mitochondria, and our metabolism gets worse – so we *DIET* again!

When we *DIET*, we usually lose muscle, lose mitochondria, and damage our metabolism. Cutting off a leg would almost be healthier. It's not about dieting to lose weight! Repairing metabolism and gaining muscle is what works and lasts.

The combination of dieting, biologic aging, and inactivity is a killer trio that sets us up for accelerated aging and falling apart.

This is what it looks like:

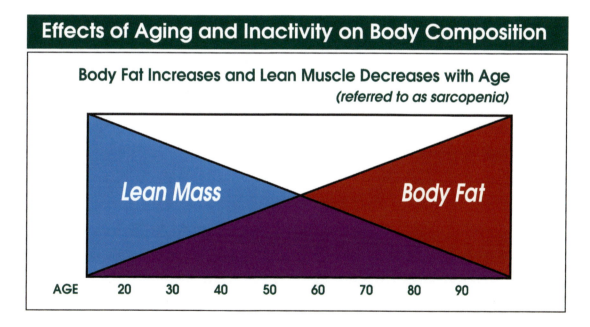

This is what it takes to reverse muscle loss, boost your metabolism, and lower your biologic age (age at which your body works):

Fitness: 3 Components

- Aerobic – cardiovascular conditioning
- Strength
- Flexibility

We need all three. The one that typically gets shortchanged is strength or resistance/weight training.

Let's Start with Aerobic Exercise

- Oxygen supply to muscle is constant
- Exercise within target heart rate range
  - 220 – Age = max heart rate
  - 180 – Age = target heart range
- Walking, hiking, swimming, cycling, rowing, running.

Many times we get on a treadmill, exercise bike, or walking track and plod along at the same pace for an hour or more - not very effective.

No wonder why we aren't fond of exercise! This is what works:

How to Perform Interval Exercises

1. Warm up for three to five minutes.
2. Go all out, as hard as you can, for 30 seconds.
3. Recover for 90 seconds.
4. Start with two or three repetitions but work your way up to seven more times for a total of eight repetitions.

Cool down for a few minutes afterwards by cutting down your intensity by 50 to 80 percent.

You only need **2X/week 20 minutes each session to boost your metabolism and cardiovascular conditioning.**

Notice that you can make a big difference in just 40 minutes per week!

For those who need something less rigorous, we have the "light version"

How to Perform Interval "Light" Exercises

- 3 Minutes walking to warm-up.
- 30 seconds – intense
  - Walk fast enough/incline to be out of breath
- 90 seconds –walk slow & get breath back
- Repeat 1-3 cycles gradually increase to 8 cycles.

Now, the most neglected and perhaps the most important part of fitness for many:

Strength Training

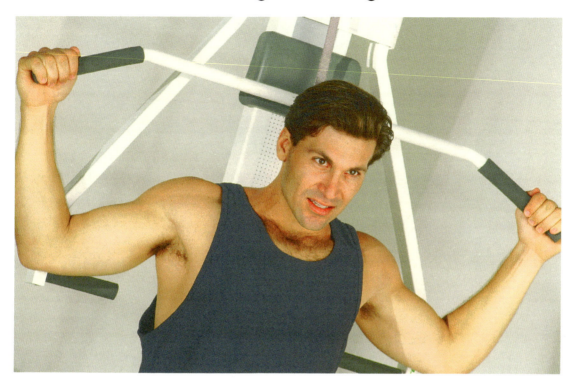

Resistance or strength training:

- Increases lean body mass – help us to build muscle
- Improves basal metabolic rate
- Helps us stay youthful and free of falls and injury

Key points to remember:

- Exercise muscle until fatigued
- Provide the calories and protein needed to build muscle after your strength training

There are many approaches that work:

- Body weight exercise (need no equipment).
- Exercise bands
- Hand weights
- Exercise machines in a gym (or home gym)
- Free weights
- Russian Kettlebells – my favorite - demonstrated in the following picture.

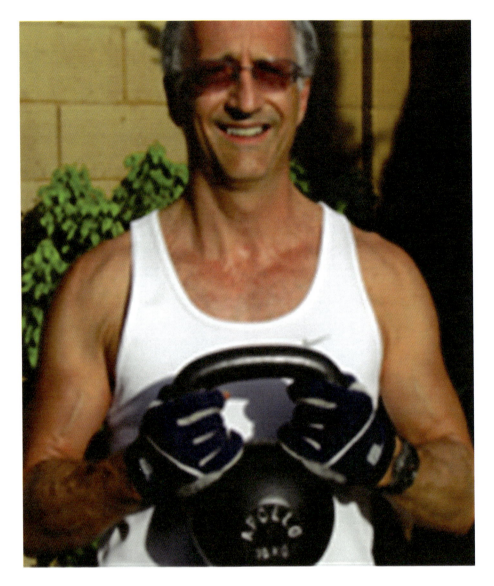

The key is to get evaluated by a qualified trainer to assess your need. Some of your muscles are ok, some are weak, and some aren't even "switched on". A skilled trainer uses this evaluation to create a safe, effective program so you stay motivated, avoid injury, and enjoy the satisfaction of looking and feeling better as you reduce your biologic age.

Your trainer can show you how to do your resistance exercise safely and empower you to do them properly on your own as desired. Others, like me, find working with a trainer keeps me motivated, improving is muscle mass and strength, and makes exercise fun.

Last, but not least:

Stretching

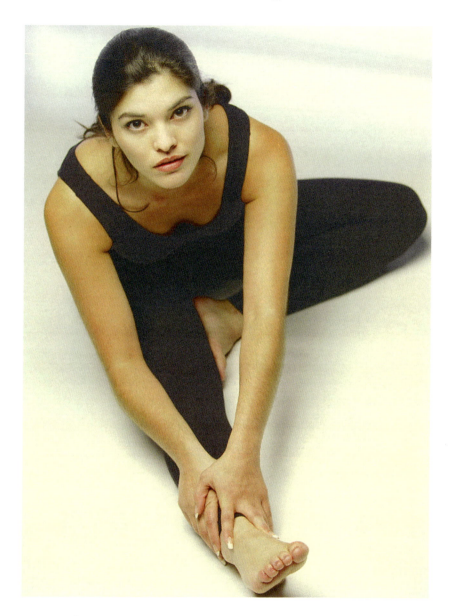

Stretching improves flexibility and becomes especially important as we get older. Older does not have to mean loss of flexibility – it just takes extra stretching and activity. The benefits are:
- Lengthens muscles
- Strengthens tendons and ligaments
- Prevents injury
- Mentally relaxing

Types of Stretching

1. Static Stretching
    a. Holding a stretch position for 30 seconds or longer.
    b. Do only when muscle is warm like *after* your exercise or after a hot bath, shower, or sauna.
    c. May aggravate joint problems if you have joint inflammation or damage.

2. Dynamic Stretching
    a. Moving a joint in full range of motion.
    b. Ideal to do as a warm-up before exercise or activity.
    c. Safer and healthier for inflamed or damaged joints as long as you only move in your pain-free range of motion.

For many, dynamic stretching is even more effective than static stretching. Dynamic stretching uses the major muscle around a joint to move the joint in full range of motion. Dynamic stretching of the hip involves swinging one leg with knee straight from front to back as high as possible for 30 seconds. Your support leg (the one you are standing on) needs to be slightly bent to avoid strain on your low back.

Dynamic stretching has the advantage of reducing injury, increasing muscle strength, and using the contracting muscle nerve reflexes to relax and stretch the opposite muscles. It's also more fun for those who get bored with static stretching – like me.

Your trainer can design your stretching program based on your needs and show you how to do them safely so are empowered to do them properly on your own as desired.

Summary:

1. Make exercise fun or we won't continue.
    a. Walk with your spouse or friend you can visit and enjoy the time.
    b. Listen to your favorite music on an iPod.
    c. Join a exercise class
    d. Work with a Personal Trainer
    e. Watch a favorite movie or TV show while exercising
    f. Be creative!
2. Keep our goals ultra-attainable. Setting an expectation of 2 hours exercise per day will lead to burnout and giving up. Setting an expectation of 5 minutes per day makes it easy to get started and if you feel good, you may go longer.

3. What gets measured, gets improved. Whether a tape measure, strength assessment, or Body Composition and Metabolism Assessment, we need to know we are improving to stay with it.
4. The key to energy, losing weight effectively (losing only fat), metabolism repair, and successful aging is gaining muscle mass (amount) and muscle strength.
5. Nothing works better than resistance exercise to build muscle mass and strength which is crucial to repairing your metabolism.
6. You need enough high quality, concentrated protein to power muscle repair and building.
7. You need enough sleep, a healthy gut (digestive system), and effective stress management to build muscle mass.
8. Having a skilled trainer or coach is essential for most to be successful.

Secret 7

Detoxifying Your Body and Emotions

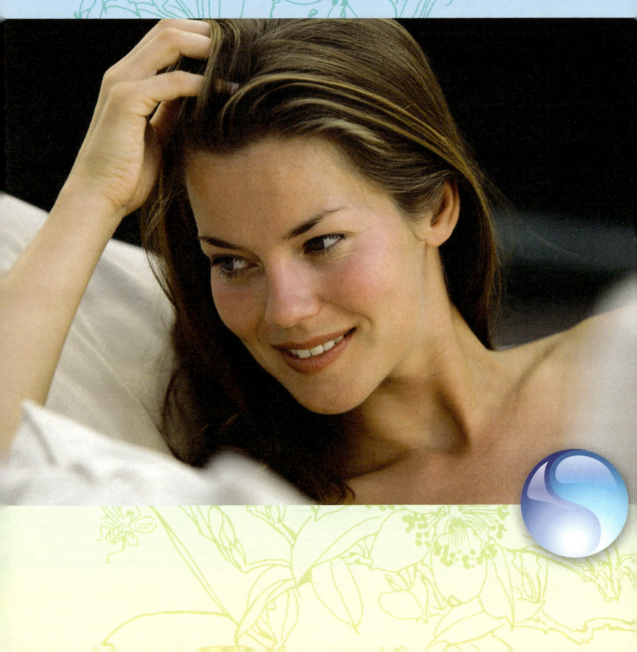

Chapter 7 Snapshot

- Toxic emotions can cripple our ability to enjoy life
- Toxic thoughts and feelings can make us sick and block our ability to heal and repair
- Toxic emotions can block our ability to detoxify toxic chemicals and heavy metals
- Almost all sufferers of complex, chronic diseases have an emotional component to their illness.
- Chronic disease is its own stressor – being unwell stresses us
- Painful thoughts and emotions trapped in our subconscious mind can create all sorts of problems without awareness by our conscious mind.
- Wonderful tools and therapies are available to help us release these negative thought and energy patterns from our subconscious mind
- Our world is becoming more and more toxic – it takes a concerted effort to detoxify and stay well
- Toxin overload is a key reason behind people gaining weight and being unable to lose it
- We can't make energy well with toxin overload.
- We have wonderful nutritional and LifeStyle tools to boost detoxification

Kate's Story

Kate came to us at age 44 suffering from:
- Chronic anxiety and obsessive worrying
- Deep, heavy exhaustion – her get up and go had got up and went.
- She had loved to exercise, now she hurts and feels worse even with light exercise – she is frustrated and worried as she puts on unattractive pounds.
- She aches all over.
- She now notices that perfumes, colognes, air fresheners, and car exhaust make her nauseous and gives her a headache.
- Some of her favorite foods now make her feel bad.

- She has been to doctor after doctor without help – no answers and the drugs made her even worse – she has spent a lot of money to get what she didn't want.
- She feels heavy and blue – depressed!

She relayed that the last time she felt good was 2 years ago. She had stressed through a very difficult and painful divorce. She had then moved into a new condo with new carpet and paint and had a full pest control spraying inside and outside her condo.

After carefully listening to Kate's story and putting together the puzzle of "Why" she has her health problems, we recommended a process to start her healing and recovery.

We recommended she start with detoxifying her mind and emotions.

Why?

Because toxic emotions and toxic thinking can stifle our body's ability to detoxify harmful chemicals and other toxic compounds.

Our thoughts and words have a profound effect on our health. When we tell ourselves repeatedly that we are fat, ugly, and will die early, our cells change to reflect this. The "skin" around each cell of our body, the cell membrane, works like the computer chip in your computer. It receives information, processes it, and responds.

This process is so profound that when you cry, the white blood cells of your immune system "cry" at the same time.

Candace Pert PhD. was one of the first to discover "Molecules of Emotion" which is also the name of her book.[1] These neuropeptides transfer our words and feelings to chemical messages direct to our cells. Dr. Candace Pert explains how emotions exist both as energy and matter.[2] Think of your thoughts and emotions as radio waves – they are electromagnetic energy – and can now be detected from outside your skull. In fact, combat helmets are in development to sense what a soldier is thinking and communicate it silently to a fellow soldier during missions.

As a practical manner, people have a hard time discriminating between physical and mental pain. So often we are "stuck" in an unpleasant emotional event – a trauma – from the past that is stored at every level of our nervous system and even on the cellular level. Dr. Pert's research has suggested that all of the senses: sight, sound, smell, taste and touch are filtered and memories stored through the molecules of emotions, mostly the neuropeptides and their receptors, at every level of our bodymind.

Dr. Pert's scientific work in the 1980's while a Section Chief at the National Institutes of Health, led to her theory of how the "bodymind" functions as a single psychosomatic network of information molecules which control our health and physiology.

We all share the human experience of pain, suffering, hardship, and trauma. We all grew up in dysfunctional homes – some more dysfunctional than others. These emotions are stored in our subconscious mind as chemical and energy frequency messages. Our subconscious mind can be a major contributor to disease and sickness – especially if it is burdened with self-sabotaging "tapes" and self-destructive messages. Our words, thoughts, and feelings have a profound impact on our health.

What is Our Conscious and Subconscious Mind?

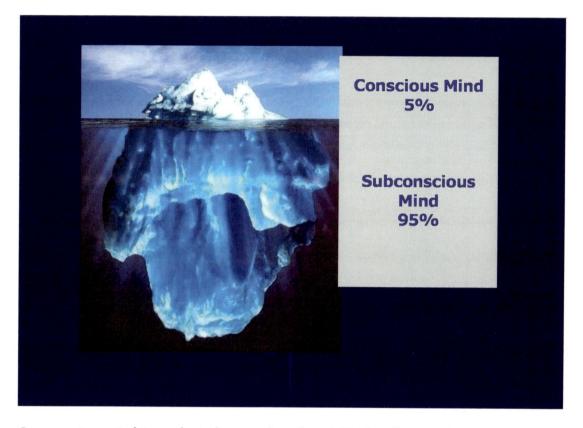

Our conscious mind is our logical, rational, analytical "thinking" part – the small part of the iceberg we see above waterline.

Our subconscious mind is our emotional, intuitive, reactive, "feeling" part – the large part of the iceberg below our conscious awareness. It profoundly affects our emotions and can sabotage our best intentions if out-of-balance.

Another way of viewing this:

Our conscious mind is the small rider sitting atop a large elephant – the elephant being our subconscious mind.

Kate has struggled with her weight most of her adult life and hated the way she looked and felt. She relayed her history of failing at diet after diet. With her logical, conscious mind, she determined she would stick with her diet.

Week 1: As expected, she did well.

Week 2: She started to slip.

Week 3: Job stress, an angry argument with a family member, and a speeding ticket would put her over the edge. She binged on her comfort foods and her diet was dead.

Why did this happen to Kate time after time even when she determined to be successful?

Her elephant (emotional subconscious mind) wanted to continue eating her comfort foods and doing what felt good in the short term and hated dieting.

She had powerful tapes playing in her subconscious mind with messages like:

- It's only a hot fudge sundae – I will only do this once.
- I have had a crappy day and I deserve to treat myself just this once.
- I need this and will feel better after.
- I am a loser – why even try?
- I am worthless and unlovable.
- I don't deserve to look and feel good.

She had plenty of emotional baggage sabotaging her best efforts.

Why?

Her rider (logical conscious mind) tried to force her elephant (emotional, subconscious mind) on a new path – the hated diet. Her rider became tired (week 2), then exhausted (week 3) – will power is a limited resource! The added stress of week 3 put her over the edge.

So how can Kate release her subconscious, self-sabotaging thought and behavior patterns so she can be free to succeed?

We referred Kate for Emotional Release Therapy (ERT)

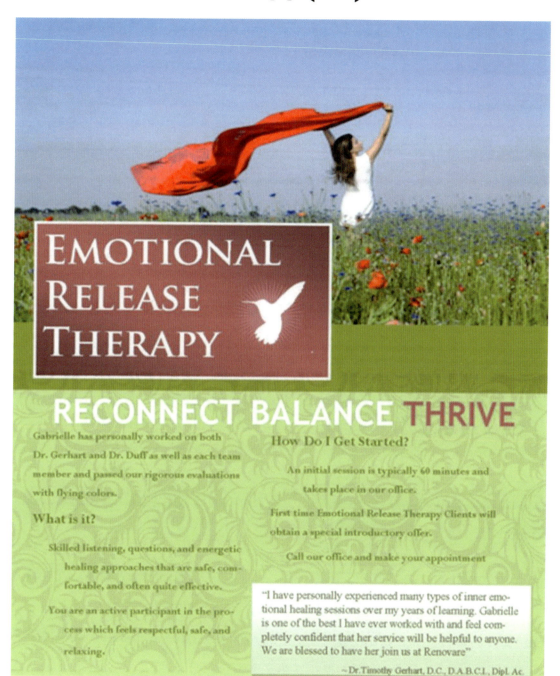

Kate had her introductory session of Emotional Release Therapy (ERT) to help release her negative emotional energy patterns from her subconscious mind. She told her ERT coach that she wanted freedom from her chronic anxiety, worrying, and emotional binge eating problems. She especially wanted freedom from her self-sabotaging behavior patterns that have troubled and frustrated her best intentions time and time again. Her ERT coach explained that ERT is an energy therapy process that releases negative emotions and energetic thought patterns from her subconscious mind. This supports healing, detoxification, and a return to Wellness.

Kate experienced lots of encouraging progress during her initial 4 sessions. After 8 sessions she hit a plateau.

I visited with Kate to get a better idea of how best to help her and referred her to our Clinical Hypnotherapist for Guided Mental Relaxation.

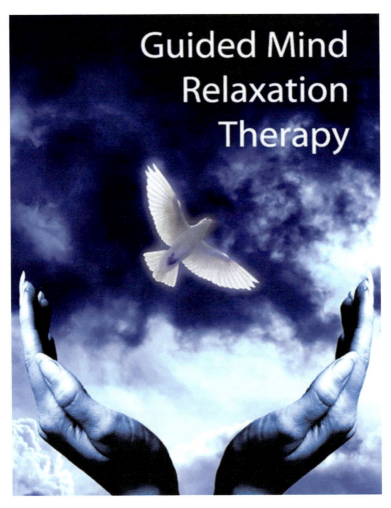

This did just what we had hoped by taking Kate to the next level. After 6 sessions and a customized CD to guide Kate into a deeply relaxed, peaceful, wonderful place and load the empowering affirmations of her value, worth, beauty, and being worthy of love. Kate was now accessing more and more of her subconscious mind and ready to take on the next part of her journey to Wellness – detoxifying her body.

Detoxifying Our Body

Goals of Effective Detoxification:
- Boost Detoxification & Cleansing
- Increase my Energy & Stamina
- Promote Muscle Gain, Fat Loss
- Reduce my Food Cravings
- Clear up Skin & Digestive Problems
- Relieve Aches & Pains
- Slow Down Biological Aging

Toxins poison our cellular engines so we can't make energy well. They trigger oxidative stress, inflammation so we ache and feel "yukky". Instead of calories from our food going to make energy, muscle, and repair us, many are shunted to storage as fat. We call this "Switched Metabolism". This is what it looks like:

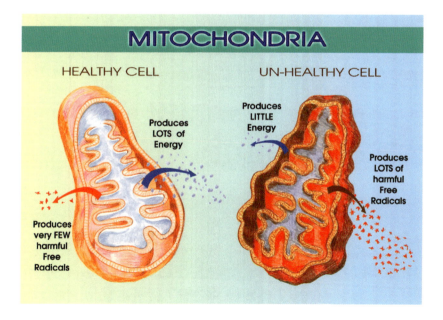

The powerhouses of each cell in your body are the mitochondria pictured above. When they work efficiently (like the picture above on the left), they generate your body weight of ATP (your energy source) everyday. They generate very few damaging free radicals.

When you are toxic, our mitochondria become damaged, biologically aged, and distressed leading to much less energy produced and many more damaging free radicals. This results in:

- You gain fat and lose muscle.
- Dieting and exercise don't work well to help.
- You ache and are tired.
- Your brain doesn't work right – brain fog – and your emotions are all over the map.

So how do we help Kate detoxify? A wise mentor, Dr. Sid Baker, states, "Get rid of the bad stuff and add the good stuff to get well". I like to think of healthy detoxification as:

Detoxification Balance

1. Reduce "bad stuff" load coming in.
   - Drugs
   - Carcinogens
   - Hormones
   - Toxic chemicals
   - Toxic Emotions
2. Increase "bad stuff" going out.

This is more challenging than most of us imagine

Our World Is Toxic

- According to the EPA, in 2000 over 4 billion pounds of chemicals were released into the ground
- 260 million pounds of chemicals were discharged into our water
- 2 billion pounds pumped into our air
- Average American consumes 124 lbs. of food additives/year
- 2.5 billion pounds of pesticides/herbicides dumped on crops, lawns, fields, and forests
- 7 lbs. of pesticides and herbicides per American per year

We struggle with toxic food, water, and air. It takes focused effort to manage our detoxification challenges in our toxic world.

The primary organ for detoxification is our liver. This profoundly important 3 stage process is :
- Phase 1 Detoxification: Occurs in our liver cells and the cells that line our intestines
- Phase 2 Detoxification: Occurs in our liver cells and friendly bacteria in our gut
- Phase 3 Detoxification: Final transport of toxins through our intestines and bowel movements as well as through our kidneys and urination. We also transport toxins through our skin and lungs through breath exhalation.

This is the reason we smell bad when we are toxic – our skin and our breath are passing toxins. This is the reason for constipation being so harmful and toxic.

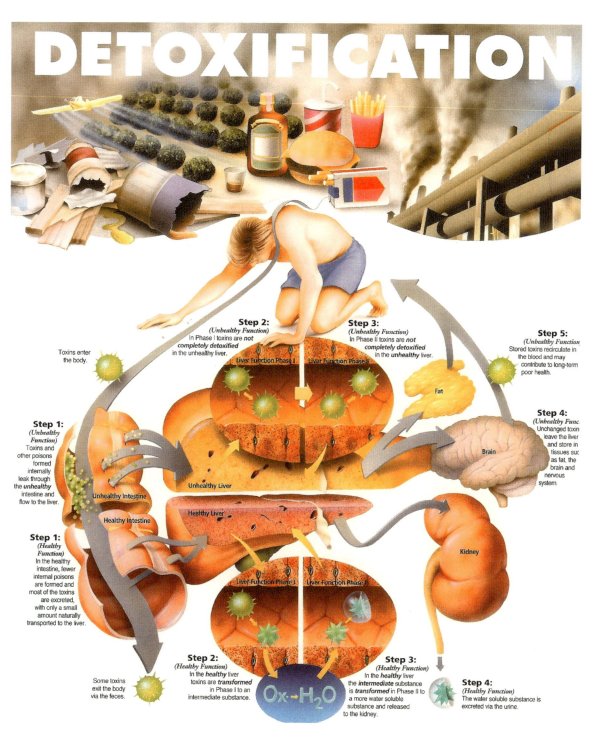

Graphic kindly provided by Metagenics

The combination of toxins from leaky gut (previous page upper half of graphic) and toxins from our outside environment add up to toxin overload. We call these people the "walking wounded" – not sick enough to be in a hospital and yet not well. How well we supply the nutrients, energy, and co-factors needed to power our liver detoxification pathways determines to a large degree our energy, metabolism, and Wellness.

The double whammy of the Standard American Diet (SAD diet) is the high load of toxins combined with the deficiency of nutrients and co-factors needed for detoxifying the junk food we eat. The nutrients mentioned below are rich in the fresh, unprocessed foods of color – especially vegetables. Another reason to **Eat Smart** as described in Chapter 5.

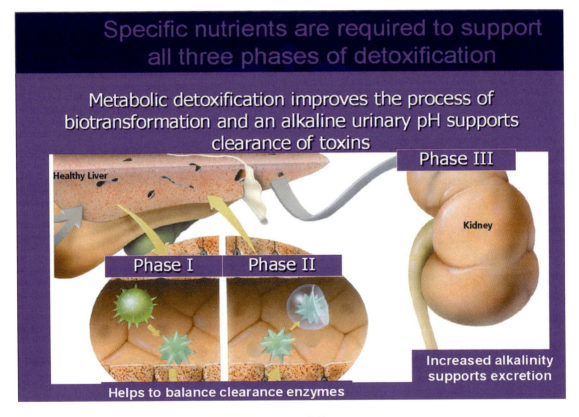

Graphic kindly provided by Metagenics

Toxins from a healthy gut (previous page lower half of graphic and in the graphic above) are processed in the liver through Step 2 (Phase 1 Liver Detox) and then Step 3 (Phase 2 Liver Detox) and then eliminated from our bodies by Step 4 (Phase 3 Detox).

The following 3 graphics show Phase 1, 2, and 3 Detoxification in more detail. In patients suffering with chronic disease, fatigue and chemical sensitivity, we typically find poor Phase 2 Detoxification and depleted antioxidants – especially glutathione.

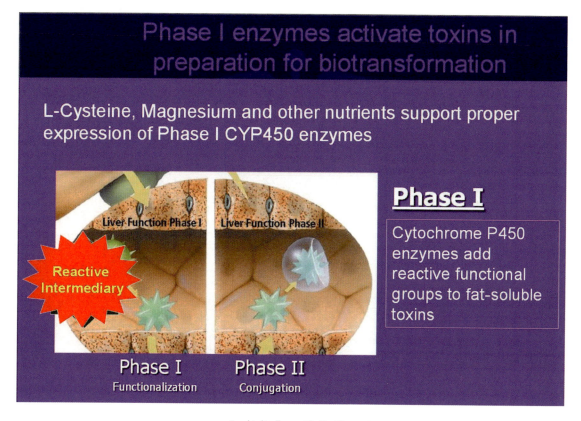

Graphic kindly provided by Metagenics

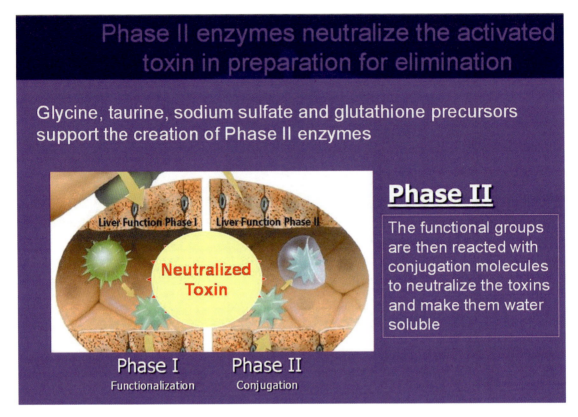

Graphic kindly provided by Metagenics

People often ask for a "Detox Program". Since everyone is different, our Detox Program must fit our unique needs and we need ways to measure effectiveness. We have testing from in-depth to budget-friendly to do just this. The Body Composition and Metabolism Assessment from Chapter 1 is one of my favorite tools for monitoring toxic load.

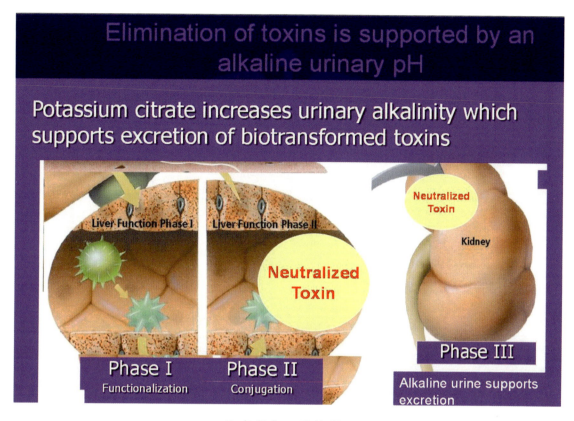

Graphic kindly provided by Metagenics

When we did Kate's blood lab Wellness Panel, we uncovered evidence of genetic "weak" spots in her Phase 2 detoxification. We used physician-grade supplements designed to support Phase 2 detoxification that work great to help correct this. Some of my favorites are:
- Clear Boost Pro to support the liver detoxification pathways and alkalize the urine to support excretion.
- DetoxClear Pro to specifically support Phase 2 liver detoxification.

We recommended a NSF tested and validated, high-grade water filter for her sink and fridge that is budget-friendly and easy to maintain(see Multipure Water Filtration in Resource Section). We taught her how to use eco-friendly cleaning chemicals, laundry detergents, and cosmetics. We also referred her to an organic pest control service.

How did Kate do?

Her LifeStyle score improved from the "terrible" range to the "looking good" range. Her energy more than doubled, she has gained muscle, lost over 20 pounds of body fat, fits into her "thin person" clothes and is enjoying life for the first time in years.

She looks great, feels great, and is happy and peaceful. Most importantly, Kate feels special, significant, and worthy of being loved. She is well on her journey toward true Wellness.

Summary:

- Toxic emotions can cripple our ability to enjoy life
- Toxic thoughts and feelings can make us sick and block our ability to heal and repair
- Toxic emotions can block our ability to detoxify toxic chemicals and heavy metals
- Almost all sufferers of complex, chronic diseases have an emotional component to their illness.
- Chronic disease is its own stressor – being unwell stresses us
- Painful thoughts and emotions trapped in our subconscious mind can create all sorts of problems without awareness by our conscious mind.
- Wonderful tools and therapies are available to help us release these negative thought and energy patterns from our subconscious mind
- Our world is becoming more and more toxic – it takes a concerted effort to detoxify and stay well
- Toxin overload is a key reason behind people gaining weight and being unable to lose it
- We can't make energy well with toxin overload.
- We have wonderful nutritional and LifeStyle tools to boost detoxification – and the tools to measure the effectiveness of your detoxification.

How Do I Get Started?

Step 1: Take responsibility for your current health. For the most part, your current level of health, or lack of, is the result of your LifeStyle choices.

Step 2: Clarify your motivating health goals. When your motivation is strong enough, you can do almost anything. An impotent goal like "Lose weight" has almost no chance for success. A goal of "I want to become lean, trim, and fit by repairing my metabolism so that I gain muscle and lose belly fat easily so that I never need to diet again and can fit into my fun clothes and look great in my swim suit for my vacation on the beach" has motivating power. You can *see* it and *feel* it.

Step 3: Repair your digestion. For some this is as simple as laying off the junk food, sodas, and taking a high grade multiple vitamin and mineral. For many, this will require an experienced health care professional to guide them through the "4R" program from Chapter 2.

Step 4: Optimize your sleep. For some, this is as simple as turning off the TV and computer an hour before bedtime and taking magnesium before bed. For many, they will need an experienced health care professional to sort out the roots of their health problems and create a treatment approach to help.

Step 5: Measure where you are at. What get's measured gets improved. The LifeStyle Score in the resource section at end of this book is a great start. Another is the "Body Composition and Metabolism assessment" described in Chapter 3.

Step 6: Improve your LifeStyle per the 7 Secrets to Wellness until you achieve your goals – and then celebrate your success!

Step 7: Pass it on! Sharing your story has powerful healing benefits for you and for those you care about. A story offers hope and encouragement for those who are ready and is just a good story for those not yet ready. It does, however, plant seeds for when they are ready. As the saying goes, "you can lead a horse to water but you can't make them drink". You can, however, give them salt through your story and example to make them *really* thirsty.

I and my team at Renovare are also available to assist you as desired. Our contact information is in the Reference Guide at end of this book.

Most of all, remember to enjoy the journey. It's all about progress, not perfection.

Resource Guide

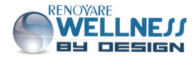

LifeStyle Score

Name: _____ E-mail: _____ Date: _____

My most important health and wellness goal: _____

_____

(Put Xs on the graphs below)

Score:

1. My food choices for the past week have been:
Junk Food <—— 1 —— 2 —— 3 —— 4 —— 5 —— 6 —— 7 —— 8 —— 9 —— 10 ——> Organic, fresh veggies-fruit, Organic lean poultr   _____

2. My weekly exercise for the past week has been:
None <—— 1 hr —— 2 hr —— 3 hr —— 4 hr —— 5 hr —— 6 hr —— 7 hr —— 8 hr —— 9 hr ——> 10+ hr/wk   _____

3. My peacefulness and emotional balance for the past week has been:
Unbearably stressed <—— 1 —— 2 —— 3 —— 4 —— 5 —— 6 —— 7 —— 8 —— 9 —— 10 ——> Delightfully peaceful and balanced   _____

4. My restful and restorative quality and amount of sleep for the past week has been:
Terrible sleep <—— 1 —— 2 —— 3 —— 4 —— 5 —— 6 —— 7 —— 8 —— 9 —— 10 ——> Deep, uninterrupted sleep-Awake rested and restored   _____

5. I have taken my nutritional supplements for the past week:
None <—— 1 —— 2 —— 3 —— 4 —— 5 —— 6 —— 7 —— 8 —— 9 —— 10 ——> As recommended every day.   _____

6. My sufficient daily pure water intake for the past week has been:
None: <—— 1 —— 2 —— 3 —— 4 —— 5 —— 6 —— 7 —— 8 —— 9 —— 10 ——> 3 or more liters/day   _____

7. I have had Bowel Movements (without laxatives or help) during the past week:
0<———— 1 ———— 2 ———— 7 ———— 9 ———— 10 ———— 7 ———— 4 ———— 3 ———— 2 ————>0
Too few 1-2/wk   3-4/wk   5-6/wk   Daily   2/day   Ideal 3/day   4/day   5/day   6/day   7/day   8/day-Too frequent   _____

8. My energy and stamina level for the past week has been:
Terrible <—— 1 —— 2 —— 3 —— 4 —— 5 —— 6 —— 7 —— 8 —— 9 —— 10 ——> Satisfied/Delighted   _____

9. My focus/concentration and memory for the past week has been:
Terrible <—— 1 —— 2 —— 3 —— 4 —— 5 —— 6 —— 7 —— 8 —— 9 —— 10 ——> Satisfied/Delighted   _____

10. My body weight and leanness is:
Terrible <—— 1 —— 2 —— 3 —— 4 —— 5 —— 6 —— 7 —— 8 —— 9 —— 10 ——> Satisfied/Delighted   _____

11. My fitness and body attractiveness is:
Terrible <—— 1 —— 2 —— 3 —— 4 —— 5 —— 6 —— 7 —— 8 —— 9 —— 10 ——> Satisfied/Delighted   _____

12. My digestion for the past week has been:
Terrible <—— 1 —— 2 —— 3 —— 4 —— 5 —— 6 —— 7 —— 8 —— 9 —— 10 ——> Satisfied/Delighted
Gas-Bloat-Pain-Diarrhea-Constipation   Formed BM's-Gas, Pain, Bloat Free   _____

13. My sexual health, sex drive, and vitality is:
Terrible <—— 1 —— 2 —— 3 —— 4 —— 5 —— 6 —— 7 —— 8 —— 9 —— 10 ——> Satisfied/Delighted   _____

14. I look and feel younger than my age with face and skin youthful in appearance:
Terrible <—— 1 —— 2 —— 3 —— 4 —— 5 —— 6 —— 7 —— 8 —— 9 —— 10 ——> Satisfied/Delighted   _____

CONTINUE TO PAGE 2   Total Score Page 1: _____

Copyright 2009 Timothy C. Gerhart, D.C., D.A.B.C.I., Dipl. Ac. Chiropractic Internist

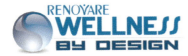

LifeStyle Score

15. My ability to be active free of muscle and joint pain or limitation is:
Terrible <—— 1 —— 2 —— 3 —— 4 —— 5 —— 6 —— 7 —— 8 —— 9 —— 10 ——> Satisfied/Delighted _____

16. My Body Detoxification and Low-Toxic LifeStyle is
Terrible <—— 1 —— 2 —— 3 —— 4 —— 5 —— 6 —— 7 —— 8 —— 9 —— 10 ——> Satisfied/Delighted _____

17. My hormonal balance and health is.
Terrible <—— 1 —— 2 —— 3 —— 4 —— 5 —— 6 —— 7 —— 8 —— 9 —— 10 ——> Satisfied/Delighted _____

18. How I feel about my LifeStyle improvement process.
Terrible <—— 1 —— 2 —— 3 —— 4 —— 5 —— 6 —— 7 —— 8 —— 9 —— 10 ——> Satisfied/Delighted _____

19. My Waist _____ My Hips _____   (W/H = _____)
Calculated by Certified Lifestyle Professional

	1	2	3	4	5	6	7	8	9	10
Terrible <										> Excellent
	>1.0	0.9	0.85		0.8		0.75		0.7	<0.65 FEMALE
	>1.2	1.1	1.05		1.0		0.95		0.9	<0.85 MALE

_____

How to Calculate Waist Hip Ratio

Waist Hip Ratio is calculated by dividing the measurement of your waist by the measurement of your hips.

How to Get Your Waist and Hip Measurements

Use a measuring tape to take your waist and hip measurement. If you do not have a measuring tape available, use a long piece of string instead and then measure the length of the string against a flat ruler.

Stand in a relaxed position breathing normally when you take the measurement. Do not pull tightly on the measuring tape or string.

Waist: Your waist measurement should be taken at the smaller section of your natural waist, usually located just above the belly button.

Hips: Your hip measurement should be taken at the your hips on the widest part of your buttocks.

Total Score Page 2: _____

Total Score Page 1: _____

Total LifeStyle Score: _____

My Total Score

150+	Having Fun Now – I Rock!
135 – 149	Looking Pretty Good
120 – 134	I'm On My Way
100 – 119	I Need Work
85 – 99	Could Be Better
< 85	My Life Style Is Terrible – When Is Now A Time To Change?

Copyright 2009 Timothy C. Gerhart, D.C., D.A.B.C.I., Dipl. Ac. Chiropractic Internist

My 7 Day Meal Plan

<u>Monday and Friday</u>

Breakfast:
- Protein: 1-2 servings
- Vegetable or Fruit:
- Starchy Carb Source:

Mid-AM snack

Lunch:
- Protein: 1-2 servings
- Vegetable or Fruit:
- Starchy Carb Source:

Dinner:

Mid-PM snack
- Protein: 1 serving
- Vegetable or Fruit:
- Starchy Carb Source:

<u>Tuesday and Saturday</u>

Breakfast:
- Protein: 1-2 servings
- Vegetable or Fruit:
- Starchy Carb Source:

Mid-AM snack

Lunch:
- Protein: 1-2 servings
- Vegetable or Fruit:
- Starchy Carb Source:

Dinner:

Mid-PM snack
- Protein: 1 serving
- Vegetable or Fruit:
- Starchy Carb Source:

Wednesday and Sunday

Breakfast:
- Protein: 1-2 servings
- Vegetable or Fruit:
- Starchy Carb Source:

Mid-AM snack:

Lunch:
- Protein: 1-2 servings
- Vegetable or Fruit:
- Starchy Carb Source:

Dinner:
- Protein: 1 serving
- Vegetable or Fruit:
- Starchy Carb Source:

Mid-PM snack:

Thursday

Breakfast:
- Protein: 1-2 servings
- Vegetable or Fruit:
- Starchy Carb Source:

Mid-AM snack

Lunch:
- Protein: 1-2 servings
- Vegetable or Fruit:
- Starchy Carb Source:

Mid-PM snack

Dinner: 1 serving
- Protein:
- Vegetable or Fruit:
- Starchy Carb Source:

Food List – Protein and Veggies

Concentrated Proteins – 15 gram serving size:

- Grass-fed, Organic, or Natural Beef – lean best 2 oz.
- Antibiotic-free or Organic Pork – 2 oz.
- Buffalo, Elk, Venison or other wild game meat. 2 oz.
- Organic or free-range, antibiotic-free, hormone-free Chicken 2 oz.
- Organic or free-range, antibiotic-free, hormone-free Turkey 2 oz.
- Alaskan wild caught Salmon – fresh, frozen, canned. (Note avoid Tuna due to mercury contamination)
- Alaskan wild caught halibut, cod, mackerel, trout (cold water fish family) 3 oz. See vitalchoice.com for online frozen shipped to your home.
- Organic Eggs – 2 lg.
- Organic Soy/Legumes: beans, tofu, lentils 6oz
- Complete Boost Pro – 1.5 scoops
- Lean Boost Pro – 2 scoops
- Ultrameal bar – 1 bar

Non-Starchy Vegetables — *minimum* of 3-4 servings per day (1 serving = ½ cup):

- Artichokes
- Asparagus
- Bamboo shoots
- Bean sprouts
- Bell or other peppers
- Broccoli
- Brussel Sprouts
- Cabbage (all types)
- Cauliflower
- Celery
- Chives, onion, leeks
- Cucumber/dill pickles
- Eggplant
- Greens: bok choy, escarole, Swiss chard, spinach, mustard/beet greens, lettuce
- Green beans
- Mushrooms
- Radishes
- Salsa
- Sea vegetables
- Tomatoes & Water Chestnuts

Starchy Vegetables – *maximum of 1-2 servings per day (1 serving = ½ cup):*

- Okra
- Zucchini, yellow, summer or spaghetti squash
- Beets, winter squash, carrots, sweet potatoes (yams)
- Yukon potatoes

Food List – Legumes, Grains, Fruit

Ideal Legumes – support metabolism & fat loss:

- Garbanzo beans
- Hummus = garbanzo bean base creamy dip – very good
- Lentils
- Pinto beans
- Black beans
- Navy beans
- Peas
- Bean soups

Ideal Fruits – *fresh, organic best, high in health promoting phytonutrients*

- Apples - organic
- Blueberries - wild
- Blackberries
- Strawberries-organic
- Rasberries
- Cherries-organic
- Canteloupe
- Honeydew Melon
- Mango
- Figs – fresh only
- Plums
- Nectarines
- Pears
- Apricots
- Peaches
- Tangerines
- Grapefruit
- Oranges
- Grapes – organic only

Whole Grains – organic best – (1 serving = ½ cup)   Note: Decrease or eliminate for belly fat loss

- Brown rice
- Wild Rice
- Basmati Rice
- Quinoa
- Buckwheat
- Gluten-free Pasta
- Gluten-free bread – Udi's or Rudi's
- Gluten-free Nutty Rice Cereal
- Quinoa Flake Hot Cereal
- Bob's Gluten-free hot cereal

Recommended Reading:

The Paleo Diet: *Lose Weight and Get Healthy by Eating the Food You Were Designed to Eat* by Loren Cordain PhD.

Dr. Mercola's Total Health Cookbook and Program by Dr. Joseph Mercola

Genetic Nutritioneering – *How You Can Modify Inherited Traits and Live a Longer, Healthier Life* by Jeffrey S. Bland Ph.D.

UltraMetabolism – *The Simple Plan for Automatic Weight Loss,* by Mark Hyman MD

The Gluten Connection: How Gluten Sensitivity May Be Sabotaging Your Health - *And What You Can Do to Take Control Now* by Sheri Lieberman PhD., CNS, FACN

Dangerous Grains: Why Gluten Cereal Grains May Be Hazardous To Your Health [Paperback] by James Braly M.D. and Ron Hoggan M.A.

Dr. Perlmutter's The Better Brain Book by David Perlmutter, MD, FACN

BrainRecovery.Com – *Powerful Therapy for Challenging Brain Disorders* by David Perlmutter, MD, FACN

Dr. Perlmutter's Raise a Smarter Child by Kindergarten - *Build a Better Brain and Increase IQ by up to 30 Points* by David Perlmutter, MD, FACN

Fast Food Nation: The Dark Side of the All-American Meal by Eric Schlosser

Talking Dirty With The Queen of Clean: Housekeeping's Royal Lady shares hundreds of fast, ingenious tips! By Linda Cobb

Recommend Websites:

www.wellnessbydesignpro.com This is our website at Renovare Wellness by Design and Clinic. To read more patient stories, go to: http://wellnessbydesignpro.com/custom_content/c_71771_testimonials.html

Copies of LifeStyle Score can be downloaded from our website above.

Dr. Gerhart can also be reached at his office number of 623 – 776 - 0206. He can also be reached at his clinic address of 18969 N. 83rd Ave. Suite 1 Peoria, Arizona 85382

Dr. Mercola's Optimal Wellness Newsletter – website, www.mercola.com Dr. Mercola provides the most popular alternative health web sites in the world and a free bi-weekly e-newsletter.

http://www.foodincmovie.com/ is the site to learn about the highly recommended movie, "Food Inc." You will never need encouragement to choose organic or free range meats after watching this must-see movie.

Recommended Products:

Wellness Meats for healthy, grass-fed beef: http://www.grasslandbeef.com/StoreFront.bok

Multipure Water Filter Systems: http://www.multipureco.com/why_multi.htm

References

Introduction references:
1. http://www.who.int/healthinfo/paper30.pdf accessed 6/10/2011
2. *JAMA 2004;292(9):1057-1059* Halsted Holman, MD Author Affiliation: Stanford University, School of Medicine, Palo Alto, Calif.
3. Circulation (2004:109:3244-55)

Chapter 1 references:
1. (1)AM Psycol, 2007 April 62(3); 220-33
2. (2)www.physorg.com/news94906931.html
3. EPA's Office of Research and Development's "Total Exposure Assessment Methodology (TEAM) Study" (Volumes I through IV, completed in 1985
4. Sources: Health Canada; BodyBurden from the Environmental Working Group study led by Mount Sinai School of Medicine; U.S. National Institutes of Health http://www.ewg.org/news/worst-families-environmental-contaminants
5. Cheng, N., The effects of electric currents on ATP Generation, Protein Synthesis, and membrane transport in rat skin. Orth Surg. 1982

Chapter 3 references:
1. Cheng, N., The effects of electric currents on ATP Generation, Protein Synthesis, and membrane transport in rat skin. Orth Surg. 1982

Chapter 4 references:
1. http://sprouts.com/ad/magazine/GlutenFreeGuideAug2010.pdf

Chapter 5 references:

1. <u>What We Eat In America, NHANES 2001-2002: Usual Nutrient Intakes from Food Compared to Dietary Reference Intakes </u>(56-page report) Moshfegh, AJ; Goldman, JD; and Cleveland, LE. 2005. U.S. Department of Agriculture, Agricultural Research Service

2. <u>'Increasing longevity by tuning up metabolism.' EMBO Rep. 2005 July; 6(S1): S20–S24.</u>Published 2005

3. <u>Vitamins for Chronic Disease Prevention in Adults, Clinical Applications</u> Robert H. Fletcher, MD,MSc; Kathleen M. Fairfield, MD,DrPH. JAMA. 2002;287:3127-3129. Published 19 June 2002 adapted from Wikipedia

4. <u>Eat Right and Take a Multivitamin</u> NEJM, Volume 338:1060-1061, April 9, 1998, Number 15. Published 9 April 1998 <u>Adapted from Wikipedia</u>

5. <u>10.1073/pnas.131195198</u>*PNAS* <u>June 19, 2001 vol. 98 no. 13 7510-7515</u>

6. <u>fishoilsafety.com</u>

7. <u>http://org2.democracyinaction.org/o/6491/p/salsa/web/common/public/index.sjs</u>

8. AntiCancer Research 31: 607-612

9. "Quantitative Factors Regarding Magnesium Status in the Modern-Day World", Magnesium 1 (1982):3-15

10. Arunachalam, K., et al. Enhancement of natural immune function by dietary consumption of Bifidobacterium lactis (HN019). Eur. J. Clin. Nutr. 2000 Mar;54:263-267. [PMID: 10713750]

11. Gill, H. S., et al. Enhancement of natural and acquired immunity by Lactobacillus rhamnosus (HN001), Lactobacillus acidophilus (HN017) and Bifidobacterium lactis (HN019). Br. J. Nutr. 2000 Feb;83:167-176. [PMID: 10743496]

12. Gopal, P., et al. Effects of the consumption of Bifidobacterium lactis HN019 (DR10TM) and galacto-oligosaccharides on the microflora of the gastrointestinal tract in human subjects. Nutr. Res. 2003;23:1313-1328

13. McFarland LV. Systematic review and meta-analysis of Saccharomyces boulardii in adult patients. World J Gastroenterol. 2010 May 14;16(18):2202-22. [PMID: 20458757]

14. Vandenplas Y, et al. Saccharomyces boulardii in childhood. Eur J Pediatr. 2009 Mar;168(3): 253-65. Epub 2008 Dec 19. [PMID: 19096876]

15. Buts JP, De Keyser N. Effects of Saccharomyces boulardii on intestinal mucosa. Dig Dis Sci. 2006 Aug;51(8):1485-92. Epub 2006 Jul 13 [PMID: 16838119]

16. Weiner, C, Pan, Q, et al. Passive immunity against human pathogens using bovine antibodies. Clin Exp. Immunol. 1999 May;116(2):193-205 [PMID 10337007]

17. Moreto, M., et al. Dietary Plasma Protein Supplements Prevent the Release of Mucosal Proinflammatory Mediators in Intestinal Inflammation in Rats. J. Nutr. 2006. Vol. 196: 2838. Robinson RR, Feirtag J, Slavin JL. Effects of dietary arabinogalactan on gastrointestinal and blood parameters in healthy human subjects. J Am Coll Nutr. 2001 Aug;20(4): 279-85. [PMID: 11506055]

18. Tharanathan RN. Food-derived carbohydrates--structural complexity and functional diversity. Crit Rev Biotechnol. 2002;22(1):65-84. [PMID: 11958336]

19. Nutr Rev 1999:57(6):177-81

20. Abraham GE. *The safe and effective implementation of orthoiodosupplementation in medical practice.* The Original Internist 2004;11:17—36. Available online at http://www.optimox.com/pics/Iodine/IOD-05/IOD_05.html. This is a good introduction to The Iodine Project.

21. Flechas, JD. *Orthoiodosupplementation in a primary care practice.* The Original Internist 2005;12(2):89—96. Available online at http://www.optimox.com/pics/Iodine/IOD-10/IOD_10.htm

22. Brownstein D. *Clinical experience with inorganic, non-radioactive iodine/iodide.* The Original Internist 2005;12(3):105—108. Available online at http://www.optimox.com/pics/Iodine/IOD-09/IOD_09.htm

23. Derry D. *Breast cancer and iodine: How to prevent and how to survive breast cancer.* Victoria, B.C.: Trafford Publishing; 2002.

24. Brownstein D. *Iodine: why you need it why you can't live without it.* West Bloomfield, Michigan: Medical Alternatives Press; 2004. Well-written and referenced, with case histories.

25. Low DE, Ghent WR, Hill LD. Diatomic iodine treatment for fibrocystic disease: special report of efficacy and safety results. [Submitted to the FDA] 1995:1—38. Available online at http://www.donaldmiller.com/Iodine_For_Fibrocystic_Disease_MX04.pdf This study makes a strong case for iodine as the preferred treatment for fibrocystic disease.

26. Adapted from www.mercola.com articles on Vitamin K.

27. The Circulating Inactive Form of Matrix Gla Protein (ucMGP) as a Biomarker for Cardiovascular Calcification Ellen C.M. Cranenburg, Cees Vermeer, et.al., Cardiovascular Research Institute CARIM, and Department of Human Biology NUTRIM, Maastricht University, Maastricht, The Netherlands; Departments of Cardiology and Nephrology and Clinical Immunology, RWTH University Hospital Aachen, Aachen, Kuratorium für Heimdialyse, Dialysis Center, Würselen, German J Vasc Res 2008;45:427–436 DOI: 10.1159/000124863

28. Food and Nutrition Board, Institute of Medicine. Vitamin K. Dietary Reference Intakes for Vitamin A, Vitamin K, Arsenic, Boron, Chromium, Copper, Iodine, Iron,

Manganese, Molybdenum, Nickel, Silicon, Vanadium, and Zinc. Washington, D.C.: National Academy Press; 2001:162-196. (National Academy Press)

29. http://www.co-cure.org/berg.htm

30. http://www.hemex.com/

31. Adapted from http://lpi.oregonstate.edu/infocenter/vitamins/vitaminK/

32. Booth SL, Golly I, Sacheck JM, et al. Effect of vitamin E supplementation on vitamin K status in adults with normal coagulation status. Am J Clin Nutr. 2004;80(1):143-148. (PubMed)

33. Corrigan JJ, Jr., Marcus FI. Coagulopathy associated with vitamin E ingestion. JAMA. 1974;230(9):1300-1301

34. Vitamin K–containing dietary supplements: comparison of synthetic vitamin K1 and natto-derived menaquinone-7 Leon J. Schurgers,1 Kirsten J. F. Teunissen,1 Karly Hamulya′k, 2 Marjo H. J. Knapen,1 Hogne Vik,3 and Cees Vermeer1 Blood. 2007;109:3279-3283)

Vitamin K References:

35. Shearer MJ.. Vitamin K metabolism and nutriture. Blood Rev. 1992 Jun;6(2):92-104. [PMID: 1633511]

36. Weber P. Management of osteoporosis: is there a role for vitamin K? Int J Vitam Nutr Res. 1997;67(5):350-6. [PMID: 9350477]

37. Geleijnse JM, et al. Dietary intake of menaquinone is associated with a reduced risk of coronary heart disease: the Rotterdam Study. J Nutr. 2004 Nov;134(11):3100-5. [PMID: 15514282]

38. Beulens JW, High dietary menaquinone intake is associated with reduced coronary calcification. Atherosclerosis. 2009 Apr; 203(2): 489-93. Epub 2008 July 19. [PMID:18722618]

39. Igarashi M, et al. Vitamin K induces osteoblast differentiation through pregnaneX receptor-mediated transcriptional control of Msx2 gene. Mol Cell Biol 2007;27:7947-7954 [PMID: 17875939]

40. Azuma K, Inoue S. [Vitamin K function mediated by activation of steroid and xenobiotic receptor]. Clin Calcium. 2009 Dec;19(12):1770-8. [PMID: 19949268]

41. Vervoort LM, et al. The potent antioxidant activity of the vitamin K cycle in microsomal lipid peroxidation. Biochem Pharmacol. 1997 Oct 15;54(8):871-6. [PMID: 9354587]

42. Shea MK, et al. Vitamin K & vitamin D status: associations with inflammatory markers in the Framingham Offspring Study. A J Epidemiol. 2008;167;313-320 [PMID: 18006902]

43. Sada E, Vitamin K2 modulates differentiation and apoptosis of both myeloid and erythroid lineages. Eur J Haematol. 2010 Dec;85(6):538-48. doi: 1111/j.1600-0609.2010.01530.x [PMID: 20887388]

44. Two-year randomized controlled trial of vitamin K1 (phylloquinone) and vitaminD3 plus calcium on the bone health of older women. Bolton-Smith C, McMurdo ME, Paterson CR, Mole PA, Harvey JM, Fenton ST, Prynne CJ, Mishra GD, Shearer MJ. J Bone Miner Res. 2007 Apr;22(4):509-19. [PMID: 17243866]

45. Ansell J, Hirsh J, Hylek E, et al. Pharmacology and management of the vitamin K antagonists: American College of Chest Physicians Evidence-Based Clinical Practice Guidelines (8th Edition). Chest 2008;133:160S-98S

46. Prevention of Osteoporosis Antonio Fernández-Pareja[1]; Elena Hernández-Blanco[2]; José Manuel Pérez-Maceda[1]; Vicente José Riera Rubio[1]; Javier Haya Palazuelos[3]; José Manasanch Dalmau Posted: 04/04/2007; Clin Drug Invest. 2007;27(4):227-232.

47. Weber P. Management of osteoporosis: is there a role for vitamin K? Int J Vitam Nutr Res. 1997;67(5):350-6. [PMID: 9350477]

48. Geleijnse JM, et al. Dietary intake of menaquinone is associated with a reduced risk of coronary heart disease: the Rotterdam Study. J Nutr. 2004Nov;134(11):3100-5. [PMID: 15514282]

49. Beulens JW, High dietary menaquinone intake is associated with reduced coronary calcification. Atherosclerosis. 2009 Apr;203(2):489-93. Epub 2008 Jul 19. [PMID:18722618]

50. Two-year randomized controlled trial of vitamin K1 (phylloquinone) and vitamin D3 plus calcium on the bone health of older women. Bolton-Smith C, McMurdo

51. ME, Paterson CR, Mole PA, Harvey JM, Fenton ST, Prynne CJ, Mishra GD, Shearer MJ. J Bone Miner Res. 2007 Apr;22(4):509-19. [PMID: 17243866]

52. Ansell J, Hirsh J, Hylek E, et al. Pharmacology and management of the vitamin K antagonists: American College of Chest Physicians Evidence-Based Clinical Practice Guidelines (8th Edition). Chest 2008;133:160S-98S

53. Barel A, Calomme M, Timchenko A, et al. Effect of oral intake of choline-stabilized orthosilicic acid on skin, nails and hair in women with photodamaged skin. Arch Dermatol Res. 2005;297:147-153. PMID: 16205932. Erratum in: Arch Dermatol Res. 2006;297:481

54. Wickett RR, Kossmann E, Barel A, et al. Effect of oral intake of choline-stabilized orthosilicic acid on hair tensile strength and morphology in women with fine hair. Arch Dermatol Res. 2007;299(10):499-505

55. Spector TD, Calomme MR, Anderson SH, et al. Choline-stabilized orthosilicic acid supplementation as an adjunct to calcium/vitamin D3 stimulates markers of bone

formation in osteopenic females: a randomized, placebo-controlled trial. BMC Musculoskelet Disord. 2008;9:85. PMID: 18547426

56. Calomme MR, Vanden Berghe DA. Supplementation of calves with stabilized orthosilicic acid. Effect on the Si, Ca, Mg, and P concentrations in serum and the collagen concentration in skin and cartilage. Biological Trace Element Research. 1997, 56: 153-165

57. Calomme MR, Wijnen P, Sindambiwe JB, Cos P, Merten J, Geusens P, Vanden Berghe DA. Effect of choline stabilized orthosilicic acid on bone density in chicks. Calcified Tissue International. 2002, 70: 292

58. Calomme MR, Geusens P, Demeester N, Behets GJ, D'Haese P, Sindambiwe JB, Van Hoof V, Vanden Berghe DA. Partial prevention of long-term femoral bone loss in aged ovariectomized rats supplemented with choline-stabilized orthosilicic acid. Calcified Tissue International. 2006, 78: 227-232

Chapter 6 references:
1. Source: Biomarkers: 10 Determinants of Aging You Can Control William Evans (Author), Irwin Rosenberg (Author)

Chapter 7 references:
1. http://www.amazon.com/Molecules-Emotion-Science-Mind-Body-Medicine/dp/0684846349
2. www.candacepert.com

Made in the USA
Charleston, SC
17 April 2012